The Science and Ethics of
Antipsychotic Use in Children

The Science and Ethics of Antipsychotic Use in Children

Edited by

Nina Di Pietro and Judy Illes

AMSTERDAM • BOSTON • HEIDELBERG • LONDON
NEW YORK • OXFORD • PARIS • SAN DIEGO
SAN FRANCISCO • SINGAPORE • SYDNEY • TOKYO
Academic Press is an imprint of Elsevier

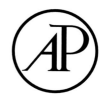

Academic Press is an imprint of Elsevier
125 London Wall, London, EC2Y 5AS, UK
525 B Street, Suite 1800, San Diego, CA 92101–4495, USA
225 Wyman Street, Waltham, MA 02451, USA
The Boulevard, Langford Lane, Kidlington, Oxford OX5 1GB, UK

Library of Congress Cataloging-in-Publication Data
A catalog record for this book is available from the Library of Congress

British Library Cataloguing in Publication Data
A catalogue record for this book is available from the British Library

For information on all Academic Press publications
visit our website at http://store.elsevier.com/

Printed and bound in the USA
ISBN: 978-0-12-800016-8

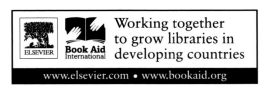

Contents

Contributors ix
Foreword xi
Acknowledgments xiii
Introduction: A Call for Partnership xv

1 A Brief History of the Science and Ethics of Antipsychotics and Off-Label Prescribing 1
Nina Di Pietro

A New Era in Psychopharmacology Research Begins 2
A Second Generation Emerges 3
The Expansion of Antipsychotics: Off-Label Use in Children 4
Benefits in the Face of Risks 6
A Call for Partnership 8
References 9

2 Pharmacoepidemiology of Antipsychotic Use in Canadian Children and Adolescents 13
Iliana Garcia-Ortega and Tamara Pringsheim

Introduction 13
Differences in SGA Regulation Between Canada and Other Countries 14
Canadian Second-Generation Antipsychotic Medications Prescription Trends for Children and Adolescents 15
National Prescribing Trends 15
Provincial Prescribing Trends 18
Manitoba 18
Nova Scotia 19
British Columbia 21
Comparing Canadian SGA Prescription Trends to those in Other Countries 22
Conclusions 23
References 24

3   Do We Know If They Work and If They Are Safe:
     Second-Generation Antipsychotics for Treatment of Autism
     Spectrum Disorders and Disruptive Behavior Disorders in
     Children and Adolescents   27
     Dean Elbe, Edel Mc Glanaghy and Tim F. Oberlander

     Introduction   27
     Methods   29
     Efficacy of SGAs for Children and Adolescents
     With ASDs   31
     Efficacy of SGAs for Children and Adolescents
     With DBDs   52
     Summary of Adverse Effects and Safety Data from ASD
     and DBD Trials Combined   54
     Discussion   56
     SGAs Included in RCTs   56
     Efficacy in ASD Trials   57
     Efficacy in DBD trials   58
     Critique and Ethical Considerations   59
     Conclusion   60
     References   60

4   Ensuring the Safety of Children Treated with
     Second-Generation Antipsychotics   65
     *Rebecca Ronsley, Lorrie Chow, Kristine Kuss, Jana Davidson
     and Constadina Panagiotopoulos*

     Introduction   65
     Side Effects Associated with SGA use in Children and Youth   67
     Monitoring the Health of Children and Youth on SGAs   68
     Guidelines for Metabolic Monitoring   69
     Recommendations for Monitoring Metabolic Changes   73
     Height   73
     Weight   76
     Body Mass Index   76
     Waist Circumference   76
     Blood Pressure   76
     Management of Metabolic Complications   76
     Why Standardized Metabolic Monitoring Matters   81
     Improving Patient Care   81
     Educating Families   82
     Overcoming Barriers to Completion of Monitoring   82
     Conclusion   85
     References   85

5   Pediatric Clinical Trial Activity for Antipsychotics
    and the Sharing of Results: A Complex Ethical
    Landscape   91
    Edel Mc Glanaghy, Nina Di Pietro and Benjamin Wilfond

    Introduction   91
    Patient Safety, Ethics, and Clinical Trial Regulation   92
    The Push for Pediatric Clinical Trials   93
    The Push for Clinical Trial Registration   94
    Reporting of Results   94
    Mapping the Landscape: Clinical Trials for Antipsychotics
    in Children and Youth   95
    Methods   95
    Results   96
    Reflections on the Current State of Pediatric
    Clinical Trials for Antipsychotics   112
    Recommendations   120
    References   121

6   Pathways to Overmedication and Polypharmacy:
    Case Examples from Adolescents with Fetal Alcohol
    Spectrum Disorders   125
    Osman Ipsiroglu, Mai Berger, Tami Lin, Dean Elbe,
    Sylvia Stockler and Bruce Carleton

    Introduction   125
    Overview   125
    Medication History in 17 Children with an FASD and Sleep
    Problems   128
    Case Vignette Demonstrating Interactions between
    Sleep Problems, WED, and ADRs   134
    Discussion   137
    Prescription Strategies and Challenges   139
    Conclusion and Outlook   143
    References   144

7   Implementing Change in Prescribing
    Practices   149
    Andrea Murphy, David Gardner and Stan Kutcher

    Introduction   149
    Pharmacotherapeutic Decision Making   150
    The Youth and Family Experience of Psychotropic
    Decision Making   153

The Prescriber Experience of Psychotropics and Decision Making   155
An Approach to Designing Strategies for Changing Prescribing Behaviors   157
Selection of Behavior Change Techniques   165
Examples of Intervention Functions and Behavior Change Techniques for Improving Use of Antipsychotics   165
Implementation of Interventions to Change Behaviors   166
Future Considerations   170
References   170

8   **Canadian Initiatives and Recommendations: Safeguarding the Health of Children and Youth Receiving Off-Label Treatment with Antipsychotics   175**
Nina Di Pietro, Judy Illes

Introduction   175
Post-Approval Monitoring of Off-Label Antipsychotic Prescriptions   176
Reporting Adverse Events   176
The ADR Reporting Process: Challenges and Solutions   177
Informed Consent for Patients and Caregivers   178
Informed Consent Involving Minors   179
Incentivizing Clinical Trials and Expanding the Knowledge Base   180
The Canadian Clinical Trial Landscape: Lengthy, Expensive, Complex   181
Becoming a Leader in Pediatric Clinical Trials: Canadian Solutions   182
Broadening the Scope of Evidence   183
Canadian Pharmaceutical Marketing Regulatory Policies   183
Industry Regulation: Policies and Pitfalls   187
Regulation in the Age of Digital Marketing   189
Helping Prescribers and Patients Stay Informed   189
Summary of Guidelines for Prescribing Antipsychotics   191
Conclusion   192
References   193

Appendix A: List of Online Resources   197

Index   201

Contributors

Mai Berger Sleep/Wake Behaviour Clinic & Research Lab, BC Children's Hospital, Division of Developmental Pediatrics, Department of Pediatrics, Faculty of Medicine, University of British Columbia; and Person Centered Medicine, Treatable Intellectual Disability Endeavour in British Columbia (TIDE BC), Vancouver, British Columbia, Canada

Bruce Carleton BC Children's Hospital, Division of Translational Therapeutics, Department of Pediatrics, Child & Family Research Institute, University of British Columbia, Vancouver, British Columbia, Canada

Lorrie Chow Provincial Mental Health Metabolic Program, BC Children's Hospital, Vancouver, British Columbia, Canada

Jana Davidson Children's & Women's Mental Health and Substance Use Services, Children's and Women's Health Centre of BC, Provincial Health Services Authority; and Department of Psychiatry, University of British Columbia, Vancouver, British Columbia, Canada

Nina Di Pietro National Core for Neuroethics, Division of Neurology, Faculty of Medicine, University of British Columbia, Vancouver, British Columbia, Canada

Dean Elbe Division of Children's and Women's Mental Health, BC Mental Health & Addiction Services; Department of Pharmacy, BC Children's Hospital; Faculty of Pharmaceutical Sciences, University of British Columbia; and Child & Adolescent Mental Health, BC Children's Hospital, Vancouver, British Columbia, Canada

David Gardner College of Pharmacy, Department of Psychiatry, Dalhousie University, Halifax, Nova Scotia, Canada

Judy Illes National Core for Neuroethics, Division of Neurology, Faculty of Medicine, University of British Columbia, Vancouver, British Columbia, Canada

Osman Ipsiroglu Sleep/Wake Behaviour Clinic & Research Lab, BC Children's Hospital, Division of Developmental Pediatrics, Department of Pediatrics, Faculty of Medicine, University of British Columbia, Vancouver; Faculty of Science, Thompson Rivers University, Kamloops; and Person Centered Medicine, Treatable Intellectual Disability Endeavour in British Columbia (TIDE BC), Vancouver, British Columbia, Canada

Kristine Kuss Provincial Mental Health Metabolic Program, BC Children's Hospital, Vancouver, British Columbia, Canada

Stan Kutcher Department of Psychiatry, Dalhousie University; Sun Life Chair in Adolescent Mental Health, IWK Health Centre and Dalhousie University; and WHO Collaborating Center, IWK Health Centre—Maritime Outpatient Psychiatry, Halifax, Nova Scotia, Canada

Tami Lin Sleep/Wake Behaviour Clinic & Research Lab, BC Children's Hospital, Division of Developmental Pediatrics, Department of Pediatrics, Faculty of Medicine, University of British Columbia; and Person Centered Medicine, Treatable Intellectual Disability Endeavour in British Columbia (TIDE BC), Vancouver, British Columbia, Canada

Edel Mc Glanaghy National Core for Neuroethics, Division of Neurology, Faculty of Medicine, University of British Columbia, Vancouver, British Columbia, Canada

Andrea Murphy College of Pharmacy, Department of Psychiatry, Dalhousie University, Halifax, Nova Scotia, Canada

Tim F. Oberlander Department of Pediatrics, School of Population and Public Health, University of British Columbia, Vancouver, British Columbia, Canada

Iliana Garcia-Ortega Mathison Centre for Mental Health Research and Education, University of Calgary, Calgary, Alberta, Canada

Constadina Panagiotopoulos BC Children's Hospital, Provincial Health Services Authority; and Department of Pediatrics, University of British Columbia, Vancouver, British Columbia, Canada

Tamara Pringsheim Department of Clinical Neurosciences, Psychiatry, Pediatrics and Community Health Sciences, University of Calgary, Calgary, Alberta, Canada

Rebecca Ronsley BC Children's Hospital, University of British Columbia, Vancouver, British Columbia, Canada

Sylvia Stockler Division of Biochemical Diseases, Department of Pediatrics, Faculty of Medicine, University of British Columbia; and Person Centered Medicine, Treatable Intellectual Disability Endeavour in British Columbia (TIDE BC), Vancouver, British Columbia, Canada

Benjamin Wilfond Treuman Katz Center for Pediatric Bioethics, Seattle Children's Research Institute; and Department of Pediatrics, University of Washington School of Medicine, Seattle, Washington, USA

Foreword

The use of antipsychotic drugs, in particular second-generation antipsychotics (SGAs), in children and adolescents is widespread in Canada and other developed nations, and has increased substantially in the last decade. These agents are used for a variety of conditions, including psychoses, mood disorders, behavioral disorders, and attention-deficit hyperactivity disorder as well as treatment of autism spectrum disorders, tics, sleep disorders, and other nonpsychotic symptoms. The use of SGAs in these populations is off-label as, with the exception of certain limited indications for aripiprazole in adolescents, their use has not been authorized by Health Canada. This is not unusual *per se*, as the majority of prescription drug use in children is off-label. What makes the situation with SGAs of particular concern in children and adolescents is (a) the range of serious or potentially serious adverse effects that are associated with their use, and (b) the lack of hard evidence for their efficacy. In particular, the metabolic and cardiovascular adverse effects associated with the use of SGAs raise serious clinical and ethical questions. These questions are especially pertinent when considering their use in vulnerable populations. This book, which contains a series of excellent articles written by leading authorities in their fields, provides the first extensive evaluation of this complex and important issue available under one cover.

It is important to remember that the off-label use of drugs in specific populations or disorders is not inherently wrong or unsafe; rather it means that there is insufficient available evidence to allow the regulatory agency concerned to include the indication in the label (or product monograph). The term "off-evidence" might, in fact be more accurate. This highlights a fundamental issue in the use of drugs in special populations such as children, adolescents, and pregnant women, which is the difficulty, both practically and ethically, in conducting appropriate clinical trials—in particular randomized controlled trials (RCTs). RCTs are considered the gold standard of evidence-based medicine and are essentially mandatory for the regulatory approval of new medicines. Their application in pediatric populations is particularly challenging, although detailed literature review indicates that many of these trials are carried out; indeed, regulatory agencies are increasingly mandating them as part of the post-marketing review process. In addition to improvements in pediatric clinical trial design there, have been exciting new advances in physiologically based pharmacokinetic modeling, which will undoubtedly lead to a much stronger evidence base supporting the use of new and existing drugs in these populations.

This book provides an important and much-needed resource for researchers, students, and practitioners, as well as patients and their families. The detailed analysis and discussion presented in the various chapters will inform the continuing debate surrounding the appropriateness, or otherwise, of using SGAs in children and adolescents. It will hopefully inspire further research into this important issue and ultimately support the development and implementation of rational, evidence-based policy.

Michael Coughtrie
Faculty of Pharmaceutical Sciences
University of British Columbia
Vancouver, BC, Canada

Acknowledgments

Drs. Di Pietro and Illes gratefully acknowledge NeuroDevNet, Inc. for supporting their work on this book. NeuroDevNet, Inc. is a Canadian Network of Centres of Excellence dedicated to understanding brain development and helping children and their families overcome the challenges of neurodevelopmental disorders. We also wish to acknowledge the Peter Wall Institute for Advanced Studies for funding the workshop "Deliberations on the Ethical Use of Antipsychotic Medications in Children" and the subsequent creation of the Canadian Working Group on Antipsychotics for Children. Dr. Illes is Canada Research Chair in Neuroethics. The programs of research at the National Core for Neuroethics under her direction have been generously enabled by the Canadian Institutes of Health, the British Columbia Knowledge Development Fund, the Canadian Foundation for Innovation, the Vancouver Coastal Research Institute, and other private funders.

Introduction: A Call for Partnership

Nina Di Pietro, Judy Illes

There are more than 60 years of clinical evidence demonstrating the benefits of antipsychotic medications for improving the lives of individuals affected by serious mental illnesses such as schizophrenia and bipolar disorder. The benefits of these medicines, however, are not without potential risk, ranging from mild unwanted side effects such as drowsiness to serious complications such as diabetes. For children and youth,[1] the risks are compounded by therapeutic uncertainties about their effectiveness for treatment of mental health conditions in this group. Nonetheless, antipsychotics are increasingly being applied to treat a wide range of emotional and behavioral problems in children, a trend that is causing many to wonder about how these medications are being used and prescribed. In this book, we explore the tension between the risk of treatment and the risk of illness within the context of off-label antipsychotic prescribing practices. Using a pragmatic neuroethics framework, we build on empirical research to inform best practices for prescribing antipsychotic medications to young people. This approach allows for the integration of a variety of medical, ethical, and sociological perspectives, which are ultimately needed to guide clinical practice (Racine et al., 2011).

The book is a direct product of the workshop "Deliberations on the Ethical Use of Antipsychotic Medications in Children" that we held in September 2013 at the University of British Columbia, with the support of the Peter Wall Institute for Advanced Studies and NeuroDevNet, Inc. The workshop brought together research and clinical leaders in child psychiatry, ethics, and neuroscience in a think tank setting to consider the state of the science and ethics of prescribing antipsychotic medicines for children. From it, we identified critical unanswered questions and formed the "Canadian Working Group on Antipsychotics for Children" to address them.

The Working Group weighed in on three key questions:

1. What phenomena account for the increase in prescribing antipsychotics for children and adolescents?
2. What gaps in knowledge need to be filled in order to begin to address concerns about safety and efficacy?

---

[1] We use the term children to refer to individuals age 0-12 years and youth to refer to individuals age 13-18 years.

3. What are the ethical, legal, and social consequences of increased off-label use of antipsychotic medications in young people, and where do we go from here?

The group deliberations under each question are summarized below:

(1) *What phenomena account for the increase in prescribing antipsychotics for children and adolescents?*

The Working Group recognized that the reason for the burgeoning off-label use of antipsychotics in children and youth is likely multifactorial—a phenomenon that situates itself within political, sociocultural, and economic arenas (Di Pietro & Illes, 2014). To date, there has been little attempt to study how or to what extent any of these arenas may influence prescribing practices within the context of antipsychotics for children. Evidence is mostly anecdotal and in the form of news reports in the popular media. The proposed factors that account for the increase in second-generation antipsychotic prescription use, as derived from our group discussions and supplemented by the scientific literature, are as follows:

i. *Wider availability of new antipsychotics on the market in the last 15 years.*

Throughout the 1970s and 1980s, the term atypical was synonymous with clozapine. At the turn of the millennium, however, several new atypical antipsychotics were developed and made available on the North American market: risperidone (1993), olanzapine (1997), quetiapine (1997), ziprasidone HCl (2001), aripiprazole (2002), and paliperidone (2006). Soon after the introduction of these atypical drugs, they quickly became the most studied treatments for schizophrenia and other indications (Meltzer, 2013). As a result, second-generation antipsychotic (SGA) use also increased during this time period. For instance, prescriptions in the province of Manitoba for SGAs went from 1.9 per 1000 in 1999 to 7.4 per 1000 in 2008 (Alessi-Severini et al., 2012). Prior to the 1990s, the level of antipsychotic use among children was relatively constant (Olfson et al., 2002).

ii. *Approval of antipsychotics to treat indications in adolescents.*

In 2011, Health Canada approved Abilify® (aripiprazole) for the treatment of schizophrenia and bipolar disorder in adolescents, making it the first atypical antipsychotic to be specifically approved for use in children and youth. In the United States, the FDA approved it for the treatment of irritability in children with autism as young as age 6. Growing approval for use in minors may contribute to perceptions that antipsychotics are generally safe and effective, even if evidence for this is limited to older adolescents with serious mental health conditions.

iii. *Emerging clinical trial data supporting antipsychotic use for youths outside of approved Health Canada indications.*

The empirical basis for the use of SGAs outside of approved Health Canada indications is supported by a growing number of studies that show that they may be effective for treating a variety of different mental health problems in children and adolescents. According to the Cochrane Database of Systematic Reviews, there is some evidence of the efficacy of antipsychotics in reducing aggression and conduct problems in children with disruptive behavior disorders in the short term and for treating the symptoms of Tourrette's syndrome (Loy et al., 2012; Pringsheim & Marras, 2009). Results of double-blind randomized controlled studies have also demonstrated the efficacy of risperidone for the short-term treatment of disruptive behavioral symptoms in children with autism, pervasive developmental disorders, or sub-average intelligence (Olfson et al., 2006). Although still limited, these positive early results may sway prescribers to adopt antipsychotic treatments for these conditions.

    iv. *Increasing diagnoses of bipolar disorder and autism spectrum disorders in young people.*

Mental healthcare resources for young people in North America have increased rapidly in the last 20 years and have coincided with increased psychotropic medication use (Olfson et al., 2014). According to national data, approximately 10-20% of Canadian children and adolescents have a diagnosable mental illness (Canadian Mental Health Association, n.d.). However, numerous studies have shown that rates of diagnosis for mental health conditions such as ADHD and autism are increasing (Boyle et al., 2011). Increased awareness and improved diagnostic tools for developmental disorders in children may contribute to the observed increases in mental health conditions and subsequent increases in antipsychotic use. In addition, the number of antipsychotic prescriptions ordered by non-psychiatrist physicians has grown. Several Canadian studies have shown that general practitioners (GPs) initiate the majority of prescriptions for antipsychotics in children and adolescents (Alessi-Severini et al., 2012; Murphy et al., 2013; Patten et al., 2012). This finding has led some to suggest that more consultations with psychiatrists and other mental health specialists may be needed to ensure that appropriate diagnostic assessments are being made by GPs (Olfson et al., 2014). Further research is needed to assess the extent to which GPs consult with mental health specialists when making diagnoses and when considering antipsychotic treatment.

    v. *Lower rates of acute and chronic extrapyramidal adverse effects with SGAs.*

The defining characteristic of atypical agents that sets them apart from first-generation antipsychotics is their ability to produce minimal extrapyramidal symptoms (EPS) at clinically effective doses. Thus, the perception that SGAs are safer may mitigate safety concerns and increased the willingness of prescribers to use them in children and adolescents.

    vi. *Lack of access to and availability of effective non-pharmacological interventions, particularly for people living in remote or rural areas or with limited income.*

Health administrators argue that access to effective psychosocial programs and services remains limited because excessive dollars are spent on government coverage of medications instead (Latimer, Bond, & Drake, 2011). Often, parents of children with complex mental health needs must rely upon a poorly coordinated network of psychosocial services for interventions that are chronically underfunded (Madsen, 2009). A misallocation of resources has also been blamed for inadequate community supports, contributing to an overreliance on medications (Latimer et al., 2011). Accessing mental health care for children is especially challenging in rural communities. Geographic and professional isolation make smaller, rural communities less attractive to mental health workers, who tend to concentrate in larger urban areas (Dyck & Hardy, 2013). Patients and families often have to travel great distances, resulting in lost work and wages and other financial burdens related to the costs of travel, such as gas, parking, meals, and hotel accommodation (Boydell et al., 2006). In contrast, treatment with antipsychotic medication may be less expensive for families who are covered under government-sponsored drug plans that pay for most of the costs of antipsychotic medications (Alessi-Severini et al., 2008).

   vii. *Cultural factors, including greater public acceptance of psychotropic medications.*

Data suggest that North American attitudes toward psychiatric medications have changed. Over the last 10 years, people have become more willing to take psychotropic medications for a wide variety of conditions, including relatively minor concerns such as coping with daily stress (Mojtabai, 2007). The decreasing stigma associated with seeking treatment for mental health problems, which has been especially pronounced among younger individuals, may have further contributed to the increasing number of prescriptions for antipsychotic medications for young people (Mojtabai, 2007, 2009). Public willingness to give psychiatric medications to children has been shown to be highest in instances where suicidal behavior is present or when a child displays oppositional behaviors and behaviors associated with ADHD (Mcleod et al., 2004).

   viii. *Pharmaceutical marketing, including the promotion of off-label use.*

Pharmaceutical marketing tactics such as direct-to-consumer advertising and distribution of product samples and token gifts that increase physician interactions with representatives have been shown to influence prescribing practices in favor of the marketed drug (Rhee, 2008). Since 2008, the U.S. Department of Justice has ordered a number of pharmaceutical companies to pay substantial fines for fraudulent marketing practices. Practices deemed fraudulent include the promotion of antipsychotics to physicians and pharmacists for off-label purposes in children, and the use of misleading information that overstates their efficacy and downplays their risks.

   ix. *Social pressures, including pressure from schools, law enforcement, and the foster care system to ensure that kids stay in school and do not get in trouble.*

Experts note that parents often seek pharmacological treatment for their children in order to avoid potentially negative social outcomes from problem behaviors. Unfortunately, almost no research has been conducted to examine the extent to which social, academic, and legal pressures influence prescribing practices. One study, however, suggests that hyperactivity and hallucinations or delusions are the most frequent problems for teachers in the classroom that lead to the use of pharmaceutical treatment (Epstein et al., 1991). Another study reports that physicians feel social pressure to prescribe antipsychotic medications when staff members complain of dangerous or particularly disruptive patient behavior (Pappadopulos et al., 2002). Other research indicates that incarcerated youth suffer disproportionately from mood and anxiety disorders that can lead to aggressive behavior. A meta-analysis of the research literature on the prevalence of mental disorders in juvenile detention and correctional facilities reveals that adolescents are about 10 times more likely to suffer from psychosis than the general adolescent population. The most common diagnoses found in this population are conduct disorder, ADHD, depression, and psychotic illness (Fazel et al., 2008). In a recent study, aggression was also linked with a greater likelihood of psychiatrists recommending off-label antipsychotic treatment (Rodday et al., 2014).

An in-depth examination of each of these nine contributing factors is needed to further inform the professional community's understanding of the circumstances that lead to off-label antipsychotic use. Meanwhile, we emphasize that this list is neither finite nor comprehensive. Each country has unique medical, social, economic, political, and legal systems that influence prescription decisions to varying degrees. As we learn more about the forces driving off-label antipsychotic use, we may also uncover dynamics between stakeholders and systems that further contribute to the phenomenon.

(2) *What gaps in knowledge need to be filled in order to begin to address concerns about safety and efficacy?*

The Working Group identified critical knowledge gaps that led to a list of top research priorities:

i. Continued investigation of drug safety and effectiveness for children and youth.

ii. Research on biomarker development for improved diagnosis of mood disorders in children and determination of risks for adverse reactions to medications.

iii. Development of guidelines about when to initiate and terminate antipsychotic treatment in children and youth.

iv. Investigation of stakeholder perspectives (e.g., physicians, parents) to identify motivations for starting off-label antipsychotic treatment.

v. Development of strategies to improve the availability, accessibility, affordability, and implementation of effective non-pharmacological therapies.

vi. Development of methods to promote the integration of research findings and evidence into healthcare policy and clinical practice to encourage appropriate use of antipsychotics in young people.

vii. Ethical, social, policy, and legal strategy development to move from an off-evidence to "on-evidence" framework for prescribing antipsychotics to children and youth.

Throughout the discussions, the Working Group acknowledged that a commitment from health agencies to partner with communities at all levels—schools, youth, parents, and health practitioners—is an imperative for affective practice models (Di Pietro & Illes, 2014). Several programs that involve collaborative community-based partnerships to provide effective non-pharmacological treatments and to address safety concerns through continued health monitoring of patients have been initiated at the provincial level. The imperative now is for a concerted effort to develop these programs into services that can be offered to all Canadian families. A targeted approach that includes champions within the psychiatric and medical community to affect change through policy is also needed. Key policy priorities that emerged from group discussions are the need to restrain the use of antipsychotics in the very young (less than 5 years) and the need to reduce concomitant antipsychotic drug prescriptions.

(3) *What are the ethical, legal, and social consequences of increased off-label use of antipsychotic medications in young people, and where do we go from here?*

This last, two-part question was especially challenging for the group. A diversity of views reflected uncertainties about the ethical and legal implications of off-label antipsychotic use for Canadian society and youth. There was considerable debate about efforts to introduce new legislation aimed at curbing the ability of doctors to prescribe antipsychotics off-label. It was evident from the discussions that imposing rules on what physicians may and may not do with regard to off-label prescribing might endanger patients and stymie medical practice.

The idea of imposing stricter legislation on pharmaceutical marketing practices, however, was met with varying enthusiasm. Some felt that it would be necessary while others cautioned that it would be difficult to implement given the current political environment, which fosters a reluctance to impose restrictions on profitable industries. Others suggested that greater impact might be had if continuing medical education courses were made available and if medical schools were required to provide more training on best practices for off-label prescription of psychotropic medications for youth. The discussion highlighted the need for health policy research to determine the best approach to changing prescription practices.

Moving Forward

This book was borne out of the need to further inform deliberations on these difficult questions. We do not claim to have all the answers or definitive remedies to the ethical issues outlined within these pages. Instead, our main goal is to provide background about the issue and insights to move forward and to open the discussion with the general public. In the pages that follow, members from the Working Group review the data on prescribing practices for antipsychotic medications in Canadian youth, describe best practices for screening and monitoring health, examine data on the efficacy of antipsychotics for off-label indications, and explore ways to mitigate concurrent prescribing practices and reduce off-label use. Throughout, the contributing authors synthesize the science to consider the ethical implications of their findings, and highlight uniquely Canadian solutions to protect the health of young people.

REFERENCES

Alessi-Severini, S., Biscontri, R., Collins, D., Kozyrskyj, A., Sareen, J., & Enns, M. (2008). Utilization and costs of antipsychotic agents: A Canadian population-based study, 1996–2006. *Psychiatric Services, 59*(5), 547–553.

Alessi-Severini, S., Biscontri, R. G., Collins, D. M., Sareen, J., & Enns, M. W. (2012). Ten years of antipsychotic prescribing to children: A Canadian population-based study. *Canadian Journal of Psychiatry, 57*(1), 52–58.

Boydell, K. M., Pong, R., Volpe, T., Tilleczek, K., Wilson, E., & Lemieux, S. (2006). Family perspectives on pathways to mental health care for children and youth in rural communities. *The Journal of Rural Health, 22*(2), 182–188.

Boyle, C. A., Boulet, S., Schieve, L. A., Cohen, R. A., Blumberg, S. J., Yeargin-Allsopp, M., et al. (2011). Trends in the prevalence of developmental disabilities in US children, 1997–2008. *Pediatrics, 127*(6), 1034–1042.

Canadian Mental Health Association. (n.d.). Fast fact about mental illness. Retrieved from http://www.cmha.ca/media/fast-facts-about-mental-illness/#.VC8U1-dH1-U.

Di Pietro, N., & Illes, J. (2014). Rising antipsychotic prescriptions for children and youth: Cross-sectoral solutions for a multimodal problem. *CMAJ: Canadian Medical Association Journal, 186*, 653–654.

Dyck, K. G., & Hardy, C. (2013). Enhancing access to psychologically informed mental health services in rural and northern communities. *Canadian Psychology, 54*(1), 30–37.

Epstein, M. H., Singh, N. N., Luebke, J., & Stout, C. E. (1991). Psychopharmacological intervention. II: Teacher perceptions of psychotropic medication for students with learning disabilities. *Journal of Learning Disabilities, 24*(8), 477–483.

Fazel, S., Doll, H., & Långström, N. (2008). Mental disorders among adolescents in juvenile detention and correctional facilities: A systematic review and metaregression analysis of 25 surveys. *Journal of the American Academy of Child and Adolescent Psychiatry, 47*(9), 1010–1019.

Latimer, E. A., Bond, G. R., & Drake, R. E. (2011). Economic approaches to improving access to evidence-based and recovery-oriented services for people with severe mental illness. *Canadian Journal of Psychiatry, 56*(9), 523–529.

Loy, J. H., Merry, S. N., Hetrick, S. E., & Stasiak, K. (2012). Atypical antipsychotics for disruptive behaviour disorders in children and youths. *Cochrane Database of Systematic Reviews, 9*, CD008559.

Madsen, W. C. (2009). Collaborative helping: A practice framework for family-centered services. *Family Process, 48*(1), 103–116.

McLeod, J. D., Pescosolido, B. A., Takeuchi, D. T., & White, T. F. (2004). Public attitudes toward the use of psychiatric medications for children. *Journal of Health and Social Behavior, 45*(1), 53–67.

Meltzer, H. Y. (2013). Update on typical and atypical antipsychotic drugs. *Annual Review of Medicine, 64*, 393–406.

Mojtabai, R. (2007). Americans' attitudes toward mental health treatment seeking: 1990–2003. *Psychiatric Services, 58*(5), 642–651.

Mojtabai, R. (2009). Americans' attitudes toward psychiatric medications: 1998–2006. *Psychiatric Services*, *60*(8), 1015–1023.

Murphy, A. L., Gardner, D. M., Cooke, C., Kisely, S., Hughes, J., & Kutcher, S. P. (2013). Prescribing trends of antipsychotics in youth receiving income assistance: Results from a retrospective population database study. *BMC Psychiatry*, *13*(1), 198.

Olfson, M., Blanco, C., Liu, L., Moreno, C., & Laje, G. (2006). National trends in the outpatient treatment of children and adolescents with antipsychotic drugs. *Archives of General Psychiatry*, *63*(6), 679–685.

Olfson, M., Blanco, C., Wang, S., Laje, G., & Correll, C. U. (2014). National trends in the mental health care of children, adolescents, and adults by office-based physicians. *JAMA Psychiatry*, *71*(1), 81–90.

Olfson, M., Marcus, S. C., Weissman, M. M., & Jensen, P. S. (2002). National trends in the use of psychotropic medications by children. *Journal of the American Academy of Child & Adolescent Psychiatry*, *41*(5), 514–521.

Pappadopulos, E., Jensen, P. S., Schur, S. B., MacIntyre, J. C., Ketner, S., Van Orden, K., et al. (2002). "Real world" atypical antipsychotic prescribing practices in public child and adolescent inpatient settings. *Schizophrenia Bulletin*, *28*(1), 111–121.

Patten, S. B., Waheed, W., & Bresee, L. (2012). A review of pharmacoepidemiologic studies of antipsychotic use in children and adolescents. *Canadian Journal of Psychiatry*, *57*(12), 717–721.

Pringsheim, T., & Marras, C. (2009). Pimozide for tics in Tourette's syndrome. *Cochrane Database of Systematic Reviews*, *2*, CD006996.

Racine, E., Bell, E., Di Pietro, N. C., Wade, L., & Illes, J. (2011). Evidence-based neuroethics for neurodevelopmental disorders. *Seminars in Pediatric Neurology: Vol. 18(1)* (pp. 21–25): WB Saunders.

Rhee, J. (2008). The influence of the pharmaceutical industry on healthcare practitioners' prescribing habits. *The Internet Journal of Academic Physician Assistants*, *7*(1), 1–7.

Rodday, A. M., Parsons, S. K., Correll, C. U., Robb, A. S., Zima, B. T., Saunders, T. S., et al. (2014). Child and adolescent psychiatrists' attitudes and practices prescribing second generation antipsychotics. *Journal of Child and Adolescent Psychopharmacology*, *24*(2), 90–93.

Chapter 1

A Brief History of the Science and Ethics of Antipsychotics and Off-Label Prescribing

Nina Di Pietro

National Core for Neuroethics, Division of Neurology, Faculty of Medicine, University of British Columbia, Vancouver, British Columbia, Canada

Before the discovery of antipsychotics, the treatment of severe and otherwise intractable mental health problems relied on risky and largely ineffective procedures such as electroconvulsive shock treatment, prefrontal lobotomy, and malaria-induced "fever therapy" to relieve patients of their symptoms. The latter intervention, which resulted from clinical observations that febrile illnesses such as malaria could temper psychotic symptoms in syphilis patients, was widely popular throughout Europe and North America (Frankenburg & Baldessarini, 2008), despite reports of serious adverse effects, including death related to parasitic infection (Hinsie, 1927).

Although seemingly unrelated disorders, the development of treatments for malaria and psychosis would merge paths again in the work of French researchers attempting to synthesize anti-malarial compounds at the height of the Second World War. Since the seventeenth century, quinine had been the standard treatment for malaria. In the 1940s, however, quinine was in short supply for the European and North American Allies because the Japanese had restricted access to parts of Malaysia where it was sourced (Frankenburg & Baldessarini, 2008; López-Muñoz et al., 2005; Shen, 1999). As the war spread further west to the Pacific theater, malaria became a serious threat, and more Allied troops were said to be dying of this disease than of Japanese bullets (Smocovitis, 2003). Hence, efforts to develop synthetic versions of the active ingredient in quinine began in earnest.

Progress, however, was relatively slow, and research on synthetic anti-malarial agents continued until after the war. It was then, in 1951, that a chemist named Paul Charpentier synthesized an anti-malarial compound called chlorpromazine at the laboratories of the French pharmaceutical company Rhône-Poulenc. Although effective at treating malaria, the new compound was deemed too impractical because it also caused marked drowsiness, to the

The Science and Ethics of Antipsychotic Use in Children. http://dx.doi.org/10.1016/B978-0-12-800016-8.00001-5

point of somnolence, when administered to patients. In May 1952, it was released for clinical investigation as a possible potentiator of general anesthesia (Charpentier, Gailliot, Jacob, Gaudechon, & Buisson, 1952). At this time, French military surgeon Henri Laborit and anesthesiologist Pierre Huguenard began using it to induce a state of "artificial hibernation" in patients treated for surgical shock, using it in conjunction with an antihistamine (promethazine) and an analgesic (Beard, 1955; Laborit & Huguenard, 1954; Laborit, Huguenard, & Alluaume, 1952). Although useful as a sedative, Laborit and Huguenard had begun to recognize its potential for use in psychiatry following observations that chlorpromazine-medicated patients often became disinterested in what occurred around them without losing consciousness. Their reported observations on the central nervous system (CNS) soon prompted psychiatrists Jean Delay and Pierre Deniker to test its effectiveness at calming patients with mania and other severe disruptive and hyperactive behaviors (Ban, 2001; Frankenburg & Baldessarini, 2008). Following several successful trials, the therapeutic effects of chlorpromazine quickly became recognized, particularly for its ability to significantly diminish the "positive" symptoms of schizophrenia; namely hallucinations and disordered or delusional thoughts (Ban, Healy, & Shorter, 1998; Delay, Deneker, & Harl, 1952; Lehmann & Hanrahan, 1954; Revol, 1956). By 1952, chlorpromazine had become available in France under the trade name of Largactil, meaning "large CNS effect." In 1954, the drug company Smith, Kline and French (Philadelphia, PA) began selling it under the trade name of Thorazine to clinicians around the world (Meyer & Simpson, 1997; Shen, 1999).

A NEW ERA IN PSYCHOPHARMACOLOGY RESEARCH BEGINS

Following the release of chlorpromazine to North America, psychiatrist Heinz Lehmann, then the clinical director of Montreal's Douglas Hospital, began testing the new drug on patients with manic-depression (now called bipolar disorder), severe psychomotor excitement, and psychosis. He conducted the first North American antipsychotic clinical trials and published his seminal findings in the *Archives of Neurology and Psychiatry* (Lehmann & Hanrahan, 1954). According to his report, chlorpromazine produced impressive results, leading to significant reductions in psychotic and manic symptoms and cutting the length of hospital stays by half (Dongier, 1999). As a result of Lehmann's research, psychiatric hospitals across Canada and the United States began to adopt chlorpromazine treatment as a standard of care. In recognition for his pioneering work in psychiatry, Lehmann was made a Fellow of the Royal Society of Canada in 1970 and an Officer of the Order of Canada in 1976, and was inducted into the Canadian Medical Hall of Fame in 1998.

Rapid advances in adult psychopharmacology in the 1950s soon triggered the development of pediatric psychopharmacology research as well. Following the publication of Lehmann's findings, several reports emerged documenting the effects of chlorpromazine on children with behavioral problems. One of the first published reports was by Robert Gatski (1955). He described nine boys who "were acutely disturbed and chronically acted out" (aged 6-13 years and all living in group homes). Each was administered chlorpromazine for 3-4 weeks. According to Gatski, all showed significant improvements in behavior without unusual side effects (although medication compliance was reported to be low, as other children in the group home frequently taunted the boys by saying that they were "crazy in the head to have to take pills"). Early reports of treatment success also included children with conditions such as tic disorders, anxiety, and hyperactivity. As reported by Moyer, Kinross-Wright, and Finney (1955):

> A small group of children ... all benefited markedly. The ages ranged from 2 to 13 years. A boy with laryngeal and facial tics was greatly helped by 25 mg given four times daily. Hyperactivity associated with brain damage was completely controlled with similar doses. Another child whose numerous fears, especially his fear of separation from his mother, had prevented his attending school cheerfully returned to school one week after he started treatment. It is noteworthy that children appear to tolerate adult doses of chlorpromazine with less side-effects than adults.

Although these early studies often had small sample sizes and no control groups, the benefits of antipsychotics for treating children with problem behaviors became widely accepted and helped to ignite a new era in child psychopharmacology research and practice (Simeon, 2004). To many, the discovery of chlorpromazine is regarded as the single greatest advance in psychiatry, dramatically improving the prognosis of patients in psychiatric hospitals worldwide (Ban et al., 1998; Crilly, 2007; Meyer & Simpson, 1997). As recollected by renowned French psychiatrist Pierre Lambert (1998), an early adopter of chlorpromazine treatment:

> ...the introduction of chlorpromazine forced us to review both our thinking and our treatment procedures ... [it] brought an added dimension of professional satisfaction to our work, in that we could now assume the status of effective caregivers or, quite simply, full-fledged physicians. We were definitely past the stage of merely trying to interpret our patients' remarks ... and then, await the generally inevitable progression and outcome of the disease.

The introduction of chlorpromazine in North America also significantly contributed to the mass deinstitutionalization of mental patients in the 1960s and 1970s. No longer confined to asylums, patients could now functionally live in community settings (Grob, 1995)—although Heinz Lehmann later fought against de-institutionalization after he realized that the process was often not accompanied by sufficient community supports (Dongier, 1999).

A SECOND GENERATION EMERGES

As revolutionary as the first generation of antipsychotics proved to be, they were also controversial. By 1954, reports had already begun to surface of chlorpromazine-treated patients suffering from extrapyramidal symptoms (EPS), which included parkinsonism (tremors, hypokinesia, rigidity, and postural instability), dystonias (involuntary muscle contractions that cause slow repetitive movements or abnormal postures), and akathisia (inner restlessness) (Crilly, 2007; Iqbal et al., 2003). Between 1959 and 1979, over 50 papers were also published on the rates of tardive dyskinesia (involuntary, repetitive body movements) in neuroleptic-treated patients; prevalence was determined to be around 20%, as compared to 5% in the general population (Kane & Smith, 1982). In an effort to minimize these serious unwanted side effects, researchers worked to develop safer alternatives. It was not until the early 1970s that a breakthrough was made, following the synthesis of a compound called clozapine.

Clozapine was unique—not only did it reduce the chance of EPS, making it appear safer, but it effectively treated psychosis in patients who did not respond to previous antipsychotic medications. Clozapine is now considered to be the first atypical (also referred to as a second-generation antipsychotic or SGA) drug. Its success quickly led to the development of others. The term *atypical* arose to describe these newer antipsychotic agents because they significantly reduced risk of developing EPS, including tardive dyskinesia, and were therefore better tolerated by patients. Atypical drugs also differ in mechanism of action, by providing important modulation of serotonergic neurotransmission in addition to dopaminergic effects. Generally, most side effects of atypical antipsychotic medications in adults are mild and lessen or disappear after the first few weeks of treatment (Mental Health Canada). The most common side effects include drowsiness, rapid heartbeat, and dizziness (Centre for Addiction and Mental Health). However, it has now been demonstrated that atypicals increase the likelihood of patients developing hyperprolactinemia and metabolic problems such as diabetes, high cholesterol, and weight gain. Currently, there are seven atypical medications available in Canada: risperidone (Risperdal), quetiapine (Seroquel), olanzapine (Zyprexa), ziprasidone (Zeldox), paliperidone (Invega), aripiprazole (Abilify), and clozapine (Clozaril). The oldest of these, clozapine, remains exceptional in that it often works even when other medications have failed; however, it is not the treatment of choice because it may cause a serious decrease in white blood cells in some patients, leading to death, and requires that patients be given regular blood tests to monitor their health.

THE EXPANSION OF ANTIPSYCHOTICS: OFF-LABEL USE IN CHILDREN

Given the history of the success of antipsychotics in treating major mental illness, it is not surprising that doctors began prescribing them for the treatment of a wide variety of behavioral and emotional conditions, either with official approval from federal health agencies (on-label) or not (off-label). For Canadian drug and health products, approval for use can only be obtained from the

Therapeutic Products Directorate, which evaluates and monitors the safety, efficacy, and quality of therapeutic and diagnostic products available to Canadians. When Health Canada approves a drug for sale, the drug approval label specifies "the population for whom the drug can be prescribed, the indication(s) the drug can treat and the dosage(s) that can be administered." The prescription and use of a drug outside of these parameters is thus deemed off-label.

In the last 10 years, a plethora of studies have reported that antipsychotics are increasingly being used worldwide for off-label purposes. A recent study published in the *Archives of Internal Medicine* (Eguale et al., 2012) found that antipsychotics were prescribed off-label 44% of the time in the province of Quebec alone between 2005 and 2009.

One group that seems particularly marked by the rise in antipsychotic prescriptions is that of children and adolescents. Today, Health Canada has only approved the antipsychotic aripiprazole for adolescents to treat bipolar disorder, both manic and mixed (in 13-17 year olds) and schizophrenia (in 15-17 year olds). However, the majority of antipsychotic prescriptions for young Canadians are ordered for the treatment of other non-approved indications, namely a variety of behavioral, mood, and conduct disorders (Doey, Handelman, Seabrook, & Steele, 2007; Murphy et al., 2013; Ronsley et al., 2013). In Chapter 2 of this book, Ortega and Pringsheim analyze trends in prescribing practices. They show that the common mental health conditions in children and youth that are being treated with antipsychotics include anxiety, attention-deficit/hyperactivity disorder, conduct disorder, depression, psychosis, and bipolar disorder. Undoubtedly, many young people with these conditions have benefited from antipsychotic treatment. If left untreated, children with severe emotional and behavioral problems are more likely to be expelled from school and become involved in the juvenile justice system, leading to a lifetime of challenges (Currie & Stabile, 2006). Parents of children with conduct disorders or aggression and impulsivity that can be harmful to others are especially in need of fast, effective, and relatively easy access to mental health treatments. Under these challenging circumstances, antipsychotic agents are recommended as part of a comprehensive treatment plan for managing behavioral problems (Harrison, Cluxton-Keller, & Gross, 2012).

Children suffering from emotional and behavioral problems deserve the best possible treatment options and have the same right as adults to receive treatment with well-tested medications, with the appropriate dose, route of administration, and indication well established. Pharmaceutical treatment options for children, however, tend to be limited because there is often no specific information about a drug's safety and efficacy for patients less than 18 years old. One reason for this knowledge gap is that researchers have traditionally been reluctant to test pharmaceutical products in especially vulnerable groups. Thus, pregnant and nursing women, children, and seniors tend to receive the majority of off-label scripts because they are not included in the clinical trials required for initial approval of the drug.

Despite some degree of clinical uncertainty, medications continue to be prescribed off-label to children because physicians recognize that denying young patients access to pharmacological treatments would be unethical. For instance, almost one-half of the lifesaving anticancer drugs given to children are given off-label (Casali, 2007). Although many of these drugs have not received official approval for use in patients under the age of 18 years, pediatric oncologists who have substantial clinical experience with these medications recognize that they can be used in the best interest of these patients. Any alternative treatment might cost patients their lives. Thus, a lack of labeling does not necessarily signify that a therapy is unsupported by clinical experience (Neville et al., 2014). Nor does it mean that data on safety or efficacy do not exist. In some cases, the data simply have not yet been submitted to Health Canada for review. In other cases, data exist but are not sufficient to meet Health Canada's regulatory approval guidelines.

For these reasons, off-label prescribing is a common, and often necessary, legal practice that is deemed an issue of medicine not subject to federal oversight. Once approved for sale by Health Canada, physicians can prescribe pharmaceutical products to whomever and for whatever purpose they deem necessary in the best interest of their patients. According to the recent Senate Standing Committee report on off-label drug use in Canada (2014), "[m]any drugs are thought to be safe and effective in sub-groups of the population that were not included in early testing of the drugs. Many drugs are believed to be safe and effective to treat conditions for which they have not received Health Canada approval. Still others are assumed to be just as safe and effective in dosages different from those set out in their product monographs."

The off-label use of medications is also widely supported by the medical community because it is a necessary component of drug innovation. Although chlorpromazine was initially developed for the treatment of malaria, its use as a post-surgical sedative and as a psychiatric medicine proved to be far more valuable. Off-label drug use is especially necessary for the treatment of rare diseases where there are inherently little data to meet the criteria for official approval by health agencies. A patient without on-label treatment options can therefore benefit from innovative uses of approved prescription drugs (Senate's Standing Committee on Social Affairs, Science and Technology, 2014).

BENEFITS IN THE FACE OF RISKS

Doctors must ultimately use their clinical experience and sound judgment when deciding whether or not to prescribe a drug for some alternative use. However, without formal, structured studies to examine the safety and efficacy of approved drugs for off-label purposes, there is an unknown level of risk involved. Despite the rapid increase in the use antipsychotic medications, the majority have not been adequately studied in children and adolescents for safety or efficacy. In Chapter 3, Elbe et al. review the scientific literature to describe the state of knowledge regarding the safety and efficacy of antipsychotics used for common childhood behavioral and emotional conditions. Although there is some evidence for efficacy in treating behavioral problems in young people, data remain limited and reveal gaps in the reporting of adverse events, making interpretations of the benefits and risks of treatment challenging for health practitioners and families. For these reasons, the extent of off-label prescribing is a growing concern and questions have been raised about whether or not antipsychotics are being inappropriately used in young people (Sharav, 2003; Sparks & Duncan, 2004; Spetie & Arnold, 2007).

Especially worrisome is the limited knowledge about the long-term safety and impact on brain development of antipsychotic use in children. Evidence from animal studies suggests that exposure to antipsychotic drugs has a profound effect on cortical development (Frost, Cerceo, Carroll, & Kolb, 2009). These effects are permanent and can influence the development of the prefrontal cortex, an area of the brain critical for decision making and working memory (see Kolb & Gibb, 2011 for review). Similar to findings in adults, there is a growing body of evidence demonstrating that SGAs can produce short- and long-term adverse health effects in young patients. These unwanted side effects include akathisia (inner restlessness), suicidality, tardive dyskinesia, and metabolic disturbances (increases in fasting cholesterol, low-density lipoprotein, insulin, and liver transaminase levels) that may lead to diabetes mellitus and weight gain (Correll et al., 2009; Fedorowicz & Fombonne, 2005; Fleischhaker et al., 2007; Fraguas et al., 2011; Jerrell, Hwang, & Livingston, 2008; Klein, Cottingham, Sorter, Barton, & Morrison, 2006; McIntyre & Jerrell, 2008; Pringsheim, Panagiotopoulos, Davidson, & Ho, 2011; Wonodi et al., 2007).

In light of health concerns, the Therapeutics Initiative (TI), an evidence-based advisory group funded by the Province of British Columbia, Ministry of Health, concluded that "physicians and parents should be especially cautious and concerned when considering using these drugs in children" (Therapeutics Letter, 2009). When the decision is made to use an antipsychotic for treatment, TI has recommended that patients receive regular health monitoring to manage adverse events and adjust treatment regimens. However, a survey of developmental pediatricians and child psychiatrists across Canada reveals that health monitoring practices are not consistent among physicians due to a lack of data and guidelines (Doey et al., 2007). For example, over half of pediatric patients (56%) are not monitored for extrapyramidal signs, and there are significant discrepancies in the timing of follow-up visits (time of monitoring varied between 1, 3, 6, and 12 months). Detailed proposals for health monitoring are discussed at length in Chapter 4 of this book.

In addition to medical risks, the social ramifications of growing off-label use are unclear. Health outcomes and treatment decisions are heavily shaped by social determinants such as income, employment status, and access to health and social services and quality education, food, and housing (Mikkonen & Raphael, 2010). Recent evidence suggests that especially vulnerable children, including minorities and those living in low-income households or in foster care, are more likely to be prescribed antipsychotics (Adams, Xu, & Dong, 2009; Crystal, Olfson, Huang, Pincus, & Gerhard, 2009). Fifteen percent of Canadian children are living below the poverty line. In a study examining antipsychotic prescribing trends for youth receiving income assistance in Nova Scotia, researchers found that antipsychotic use increased significantly in Pharmacare recipients between the ages of 0 and 25 years from 2000 to 2007 (Murphy et al., 2013). Moreover, almost half of Pharmacare beneficiaries (45%) aged 21-25 years received antipsychotic prescriptions, considerably above national norms. Several studies in the United States have demonstrated that youth in foster care are also disproportionately more likely to receive psychotropic medications. Medication use is three times higher for kids in foster care than for youth living with their families, even if these families constitute low-income households (Zito et al., 2008). Moreover, the proportion of youths using antipsychotics has been increasing significantly more among African Americans and Hispanics than among Caucasians (Zito, Burcu, Ibe, Safer, & Magder, 2013).

Research is needed in Canada to determine if similar trends are emerging for minorities, such as Indigenous youth and those living in care. Approximately 30,000 Canadian children are in foster care; of these, almost one-half are Aboriginal (Statistics Canada National Household Survey, 2011). The legacy of colonialization has greatly diminished the health and well being of Indigenous peoples: suicide rates are five to six times higher in Aboriginal communities, and high rates of major depression, problems with alcohol, and experience of sexual abuse during childhood are also reported (Smiley, 2009). Moreover, Indigenous youth are overrepresented in the criminal justice system (Corrado, Kuehn, & Margaritescu, 2014) where prevalence rates of psychiatric disorders and psychopharmacological treatment are known to be high (Engel, Abulu, & Nikolov, 2012).

Taken together, several important ethical questions emerge from the social, economic, and medical literature:

- Do the benefits of antipsychotic treatment outweigh the risks for children and youth?
- Are there ethnic disparities in how antipsychotics are prescribed?
- Are youth in foster care or the juvenile justice system more likely to receive antipsychotic treatment? If so, what is the risk-benefit tradeoff? What alternative choices do they have, and is coercion to medicate a problem in these circumstances?
- What are the unique needs of healthcare professionals, patients and parents, social workers, and educators that have contributed to the prescription phenomenon, and how can these different stakeholders collectively work together to manage health concerns?

A CALL FOR PARTNERSHIP

The medical, ethical, and social uncertainties surrounding antipsychotics have created concern that young people are at risk, and parents are burdened with anxiety about whether or not they are making the right decisions for their children. Significant progress in aiding the decision regarding medication may be achieved through the development of evidence-based national guidelines for indications, dosing, and monitoring of antipsychotics. In a review of treatment guidelines for antipsychotic prescribing for minors (Kealey et al., 2014), seven key areas of practice were identified in need of further guidance development: (1) use in the very young (less than 6 years), (2) use of two or more concurrent antipsychotics, (3) use of high doses, (4) use without a primary indication, (5) use with or in lieu of psychosocial services, (6) metabolic screening, and (7) timing of follow-up visits. Until more data are available in these seven areas, consensus-based guidelines are needed.

Given that antipsychotics continue to be administered to youth off-label, the ethical imperative now favors well-planned clinical trial research in this vulnerable group under the principle of justice, which requires that social benefits and social burdens be equally shared among stakeholders (Arnold, 2001). This approach represents a substantial shift from previous practice, which tended to avoid experimenting on young populations. In Chapter 5, the state and magnitude of pediatric clinical trials for antipsychotics is characterized in detail. Here, McGlanaghy et al. demonstrate that pediatric clinical trial activity for antipsychotics has declined steadily since 2009 and encompasses a wide variety of study designs, indications, and outcome measures. Partnerships between Health Canada, the Canadian Institutes of Health Research, and industry are needed to develop a national research network focused on the unique psychotherapeutic needs of children and adolescents, leading to improved drug research for children in Canada (Canadian Paediatric Society, 2011).

Although progress is being made, considerable work remains to be done. In Chapters 6 and 7, recommendations for reducing concurrent antipsychotic prescriptions and implementing change in prescribing practices are reviewed. Some have suggested that a national body such as the Canadian Psychiatric Association or the Canadian Academy of Child and Adolescent Psychiatry should take the lead and appoint an expert panel to produce and implement best practice recommendations (Doey et al., 2007). In Chapter 8, we end with a review of Canadian initiatives to spur research and improve prescribing practices. Several regulatory gaps are highlighted and solutions are presented that will advance national policies and enable Canada to become a leader in pediatric research of off-label drugs.

REFERENCES

Adams, S. J., Xu, S., & Dong, F. (2009). Differences in prescribing patterns of psychotropic medication for children and adolescents between rural and urban prescribers. Retrieved from the WICHE Center for Rural Mental Health Research website http://www.wiche.edu/info/publications/AdamsWorkingPaperYr4Proj2.pdf

Arnold, L. E. (2001). Turn-of-the-century ethical issues in child psychiatric research. *Current Psychiatry Reports, 3*(2), 109–114.

Ban, T. A. (2001). Pharmacotherapy of mental illness—A historical analysis. *Progress in Neuro-Psychopharmacology and Biological Psychiatry, 25*(4), 709–727.

Ban, T. A., Healy, D., & Shorter, E. (1998). *The rise of psycho-pharmacology and the story of CINP*. Budapest: Animula.

Beard, J. (1955). Chlorpromazine and allied substances. *Postgraduate Medical Journal, 31*, 451–455.

Canadian Paediatric Society, Drug Therapy and Hazardous Substances Committee. (2011). Drug research and treatment for children in Canada: A challenge. *Paediatrics and Child Health, 16*(9), 560.

Casali, P. G. (2007). The off-label use of drugs in oncology: A position paper by the European Society for Medical Oncology (ESMO). *Annals of Oncology, 18*(12), 1923–1925.

Charpentier, P., Gailliot, P., Jacob, R., Gaudechon, J., & Buisson, P. (1952). Recherches sur les diméthylaminopropyl-N phénothiazines substituées. *Comptes rendus de l'Académie des sciences* (Paris), *235*(1), 59–60.

Corrado, R. R., Kuehn, S., & Margaritescu, I. (2014). Policy issues regarding the overrepresentation of incarcerated Aboriginal young offenders in a Canadian context. *Youth Justice, 14*(1), 40–62.

Correll, C. U., Manu, P., Olshanskiy, V., Napolitano, B., Kane, J. M., & Malhotra, A. K. (2009). Cardiometabolic risk of second-generation antipsychotic medications during first-time use in children and adolescents. *Journal of the American Medical Association, 302*(16), 1765–1773.

Crilly, J. (2007). The history of clozapine and its emergence in the US market: A review and analysis. *History of Psychiatry, 18*(1), 39–60.

Crystal, S., Olfson, M., Huang, C., Pincus, H., & Gerhard, T. (2009). Broadened use of atypical antipsychotics: Safety, effectiveness, and policy challenges. *Health Affairs, 28*(5), w770–w781.

Currie, J., & Stabile, M. (2006). Child mental health and human capital accumulation: The case of ADHD. *Journal of Health Economics, 25*(6), 1094–1118.

Delay, J., Deneker, P., & Harl, J. M. (1952). Utilisation en therapeutique psychiatrique d'une derivee d'hibernotherapie. *Annales Médico-Psychologiques, 110*, 112–117.

Doey, T., Handelman, K., Seabrook, J. A., & Steele, M. (2007). Survey of atypical antipsychotic prescribing by Canadian child psychiatrists and developmental pediatricians for patients aged under 18 years. *The Canadian Journal of Psychiatry, 52*(6), 363–368.

Dongier, M. (1999). Heinz E. Lehmann, 1911-1999. *Journal of Psychiatry and Neuroscience, 24*(4), 362.

Eguale, T., Buckeridge, D. L., Winslade, N. E., Benedetti, A., Hanley, J. A., & Tamblyn, R. (2012). Drug, patient, and physician characteristics associated with off-label prescribing in primary care. *Archives of Internal Medicine, 172*(10), 781–788.

Engel, L., Abulu, J., & Nikolov, R. N. (2012). Psychopharmacological treatment of youth in juvenile justice settings. In E.L. Grigorenko (Ed.), *Handbook of juvenile forensic psychology and psychiatry* (pp. 341–355). US: Springer Science & Business Media.

Fedorowicz, V. J., & Fombonne, E. (2005). Metabolic side effects of atypical antipsychotics in children: A literature review. *Journal of Psychopharmacology, 19*(5), 533–550.

Fleischhaker, C., Heiser, P., Hennighausen, K., Herpertz-Dahlmann, B., Holtkamp, K., Mehler-Wex, C., et al. (2007). Weight gain associated with clozapine, olanzapine and risperidone in children and adolescents. *Journal of Neural Transmission, 114*(2), 273–280.

Fraguas, D., Correll, C. U., Merchán-Naranjo, J., Rapado-Castro, M., Parellada, M., Moreno, C., et al. (2011). Efficacy and safety of second-generation antipsychotics in children and adolescents with psychotic and bipolar spectrum disorders: Comprehensive review of prospective head-to-head and placebo-controlled comparisons. *European Neuropsychopharmacology, 21*(8), 621–645.

Frankenburg, F. R., & Baldessarini, R. J. (2008). Neurosyphilis, malaria, and the discovery of antipsychotic agents. *Harvard Review of Psychiatry*, *16*(5), 299–307.

Frost, D. O., Cerceo, S., Carroll, C., & Kolb, B. (2009). Early exposure to haloperidol or olanzapine induces long-term alterations of dendritic form. *Synapse*, *64*, 191–199.

Gatski, R. L. (1955). Chlorpromazine in the treatment of emotionally maladjusted children: Preliminary report. *Journal of the American Medical Association*, *157*(15), 1298–1300.

Grob, G. N. (1995). The paradox of deinstitutionalization. *Society*, *32*, 51–59.

Harrison, J. N., Cluxton-Keller, F., & Gross, D. (2012). Antipsychotic medication prescribing trends in children and adolescents. *Journal of Pediatric Health Care*, *26*(2), 139–145.

Hinsie, L. E. (1927). Malaria treatment of schizophrenia. *Psychiatric Quarterly*, *1*(2), 210–214.

Iqbal, M. M., Rahman, A., Husain, Z., Mahmud, S. Z., Ryan, W. G., & Feldman, J. M. (2003). Clozapine: A clinical review of adverse effects and management. *Annals of Clinical Psychiatry*, *15*(1), 33–48.

Jerrell, J. M., Hwang, T.-L., & Livingston, T. S. (2008). Neurological adverse events associated with antipsychotic treatment in children and adolescents. *Journal of Child Neurology*, *23*(12), 1392–1399.

Kane, J. M., & Smith, J. M. (1982). Tardive dyskinesia: Prevalence and risk factors, 1959 to 1979. *Archives of General Psychiatry*, *39*(4), 473–481.

Kealey, E., Scholle, S. H., Byron, S. C., Hoagwood, K., Leckman-Westin, E., Kelleher, K., et al. (2014). Quality concerns in antipsychotic prescribing for youth: A review of treatment guidelines. *Academic Pediatrics*, *14*(5), S68–S75.

Klein, D., Cottingham, E., Sorter, M., Barton, B., & Morrison, J. (2006). A randomized, double-blind, placebo-controlled trial of metformin treatment of weight gain associated with initiation of atypical antipsychotic therapy in children and adolescents. *American Journal of Psychiatry*, *163*(12), 2072–2079.

Kolb, B., & Gibb, R. (2011). Brain plasticity and behaviour in the developing brain. *Journal of the Canadian Academy of Child and Adolescent Psychiatry*, *20*(4), 265.

Laborit, H., & Huguenard, P. (1954). Pratique de l'hibernothérapie en chirurgie et en medicine. Paris: Masson.

Laborit, H., Huguenard, P., & Alluaume, R. (1952). Un nouveau stabilisateur neuro-vegetatif, le 4560 RP. *La Presse Médicale*, *60*, 206–208.

Lambert, P. A. (1998). Chlorpromazine: A true story of the progress effected by this drug. In T. A. Ban, D. Healy, & E. Shorter (Eds.), *The rise of psychopharmacology and the story of CINP* (pp. 237–243). Budapest: Animula.

Lehmann, H. E., & Hanrahan, G. E. (1954). Chlorpromazine, new inhibiting agent for psychomotor excitement and manic states. *Archives of Neurology and Psychiatry*, *71*, 227–237.

López-Muñoz, F., Alamo, C., Cuenca, E., Shen, W. W., Clervoy, P., & Rubio, G. (2005). History of the discovery and clinical introduction of chlorpromazine. *Annals of Clinical Psychiatry*, *17*(3), 113–135.

McIntyre, R. S., & Jerrell, J. M. (2008). Metabolic and cardiovascular adverse events associated with antipsychotic treatment in children and adolescents. *Archives of Pediatrics & Adolescent Medicine*, *162*(10), 929–935.

Meyer, J. M., & Simpson, G. M. (1997). From chlorpromazine to olanzapine: A brief history of antipsychotics. *Psychiatric Services*, *48*(9), 1137–1139.

Mikkonen, J., & Raphael, D. (2010). Social determinants of health: The Canadian facts. Toronto: York University School of Health Policy and Management.

Moyer, J. H., Kinross-Wright, V., & Finney, R. (1955). Chlorpromazine as a therapeutic agent in clinical medicine. *AMA Archives of Internal Medicine*, *95*(2), 202–218.

Murphy, A. L., Gardner, D. M., Cooke, C., Kisely, S., Hughes, J., & Kutcher, S. P. (2013). Prescribing trends of antipsychotics in youth receiving income assistance: Results from a retrospective population database study. *BMC Psychiatry, 13*(1), 198.

Neville, K. A., Frattarelli, D. A., Galinkin, J. L., Green, T. P., Johnson, T. D., Paul, I. M., et al. (2014). Off-label use of drugs in children. *Pediatrics, 133*(3), 563–567.

Pringsheim, T., Panagiotopoulos, C., Davidson, J., & Ho, J. (2011). Evidence-based recommendations for monitoring safety of second-generation antipsychotics in children and youth. *Paediatrics & Child Health, 16*(9), 581.

Revol, L. (1956). La thérapeutique par la chlorpromazine en pratique psychiatrique [Chlorpromazine therapy in psychiatric practice]. Paris: Masson.

Ronsley, R., Scott, D., Warburton, W. P., Hamdi, R. D., Louie, D. C., Davidson, J., et al. (2013). A population-based study of antipsychotic prescription trends in children and adolescents in British Columbia, from 1996 to 2011. *Canadian Journal of Psychiatry, 58*(6), 361–369.

Senate's Standing Committee on Social Affairs, Science and Technology. (2014). Prescription pharmaceuticals in Canada: Off-label use. Retrieved from http://senate-senat.ca/soci-e.asp.

Sharav, V. H. (2003). Children in clinical research: A conflict of moral values. *American Journal of Bioethics, 3*(1), 12–59.

Shen, W. W. (1999). A history of antipsychotic drug development. *Comprehensive Psychiatry, 40*(6), 407–414.

Simeon, J. G. (2004). History of pediatric psychopharmacology: A brief personal perspective. In T. A. Ban, D. Healy, & E. Shorter (Eds.), Reflection on twentieth-century psychopharmacology, Vol. 4 (pp. 685–689). Budapest: Animula Publishing House.

Smiley, J. (2009). The health of aboriginal people. In D. Raphael (Ed.), *Social determinants of health: Canadian perspectives* (2nd ed.) (pp. 280–301). Toronto: Canadian Scholars' Press.

Smocovitis, V. B. (2003). Desperately seeking quinine. *Modern Drug Discovery, 6*, 57–58.

Sparks, J., & Duncan, B. L. (2004). The ethics and science of medicating children. *Ethical Human Psychology and Psychiatry, 6*(1), 25–39.

Spetie, L., & Arnold, L. E. (2007). Ethical issues in child psychopharmacology research and practice: Emphasis on preschoolers. *Psychopharmacology, 191*(1), 15–26.

Statistics Canada. (2011). *2011 National household survey: Aboriginal Peoples in Canada: First Nations People, Métis and Inuit.* Retrieved from http://www.statcan.gc.ca/daily-quotidien/130508/dq130508a-eng.htm?HPA.

Therapeutics Initiative. (2009). Increasing use of newer antipsychotics in children: A cause for concern? *Therapeutics Letter, 74*, 1–2.

Wonodi, I., Reeves, G., Carmichael, D., Verovsky, I., Avila, M. T., Elliott, A., et al. (2007). Tardive dyskinesia in children treated with atypical antipsychotic medications. *Movement Disorders, 22*(12), 1777–1782.

Zito, J. M., Burcu, M., Ibe, A., Safer, D. J., & Magder, L. S. (2013). Antipsychotic use by Medicaid-insured youths: Impact of eligibility and psychiatric diagnosis across a decade. *Psychiatric Services, 64*(3), 223–229.

Zito, J. M., Safer, D. J., Sai, D., Gardner, J. F., Thomas, D., Coombes, P., et al. (2008). Psychotropic medication patterns among youth in foster care. *Pediatrics, 121*(1), e157–e163.

Chapter 2

Pharmacoepidemiology of Antipsychotic Use in Canadian Children and Adolescents

Iliana Garcia-Ortega[*], Tamara Pringsheim[†]

[*]*Mathison Centre for Mental Health Research and Education, University of Calgary, Calgary, Alberta, Canada*

[†]*Department of Clinical Neurosciences, Psychiatry, Pediatrics and Community Health Sciences, University of Calgary, Calgary, Alberta, Canada*

INTRODUCTION

Pharmacoepidemiology is a discipline that applies epidemiological methodologies to assess medication use in populations with the purpose of supporting the rational use of pharmaceuticals to improve health outcomes (Luo, Doherty, Cappelleri, & Frush, 2007; World Health Organization, 2003). Pharmacoepidemiological studies are crucial in research to promote the safe use of drugs. Currently there is a need for more information on the long-term efficacy and safety of antipsychotic use in children and adolescents, due to their increased use for a variety of pediatric mental health conditions. Second-generation antipsychotics (SGAs) are a group of antipsychotics also labeled as atypical or dopamine-serotonin antagonists, based on their chemical properties, which include a rapid dissociation from D2 receptors (dopamine type 2) and blockade of 5-HT2A receptors (serotonin type 2). Due to the rapid dissociation from dopamine receptors, these medications have a lower risk of extrapyramidal side effects, including tardive dyskinesia, acute dystonia, tardive dystonia, drug-induced parkinsonism, and akathisia, when compared to first-generation antipsychotic (FGA) medications (Gardner & Teehan, 2010; Pierre, 2005).

Since their introduction, SGAs have led to major changes in the use of antipsychotics. Before the introduction of SGAs in the 1990s, the use of antipsychotics was largely reserved for adults with severe mental disorders. In the last decade, the prescription of SGAs for young people with nonpsychotic disorders has dramatically increased (Cooper, Arbogast, & Ding, 2006; Doey,

The Science and Ethics of Antipsychotic Use in Children. http://dx.doi.org/10.1016/B978-0-12-800016-8.00002-7

Handelman, & Seabrook, 2007; Patel et al., 2005; Patten, Waheed, & Bresee, 2012). SGAs are preferred by prescribers primarily because of the lower rate of negative neurological side effects. However, these medications are not risk free. In addition to the possibility of neurological impairments, they are more likely to cause changes in metabolic functioning that adversely affect health. The metabolic side effects include weight gain, hyperglycemia, dyslipidemia, hypertension, and metabolic syndrome, effects that also increase cardiovascular risk (Morrato, Nicol, & Maahs, 2010). A more detailed discussion of the adverse side effects of antipsychotics is included in another chapter of this book.

The increased use of SGAs is particularly concerning in children because of observed patterns in their length of use (Pringsheim, Panagiotopoulos, Davidson, Ho, & Group, 2011) and the well-known chronic evolution of the majority of mental disorders (Prince et al., 2007). In addition, the lack of systematic assessment, screening, monitoring of side effects, and identification of modifiable cardiovascular risk factors is concerning given the potential long-term health consequences (Morrato et al., 2010; Pringsheim, Lam, Ching, & Patten, 2011).

DIFFERENCES IN SGA REGULATION BETWEEN CANADA AND OTHER COUNTRIES

Most countries have a drug regulatory authority that plays a key role in the licensing process and prescriptions. Drug regulatory authorities around the world differ substantially based on their human and financial resources, making regulation of drug licensing and use between countries considerably different. Even among industrialized high-income countries the differences between licensed and unlicensed medications varies significantly. Regardless of drug regulatory authorities, clinicians are in fact free to prescribe outside the licensing term (off-license or off-label). This occurs within certain boundaries, dictated by practice guidelines based on sufficient and satisfactory evidence, and in this case the clinician assumes a greater professional responsibility.

In Canada, there are nine available SGAs on the market: clozapine, risperidone, olanzapine, quetiapine, paliperidone, ziprasidone, aripiprazole, asenapine, and lurasidone. At present, their use in children is off-label, as no SGAs have received an official indication by Health Canada for use in children or adolescents, with the exception of aripiprazole. Aripiprazole was authorized in December 2011 for use in adolescents aged 15 and older with a diagnosis of schizophrenia and for the treatment of manic or mixed episodes in bipolar I disorder as monotherapy in adolescents 13-17 years of age (Canada Adverse Reaction Newsletter, 2012). SGAs are often used off-label to treat a large spectrum of youth mental disorders, including aggression in attention-deficit/hyperactivity disorder (ADHD), oppositional defiant disorder, conduct disorder, irritability related to autism spectrum disorders, mood dysregulation, eating disorders, and tic disorders (Alessi-Severini, Biscontri, Collins, Sareen, & Enns,

2012; Murphy et al., 2013; Pringsheim, Lam, Ching, et al., 2011; Pringsheim, Lam, & Patten, 2011; Pringsheim, Panagiotopoulos, et al., 2011).

In the United States, risperidone was first approved by the Food and Drug Administration to treat schizophrenia and bipolar disorder in youth in 2007. It is now also approved to treat severe behavioral problems, including aggression and irritability in children with autism aged 5-17. Aripiprazole has also been approved for the same indications but for children ages 6-17. Risperidone, aripiprazole, and quetiapine are approved for the treatment of 13- to 17-year-old adolescents with schizophrenia and 10- to 17-year-old youths with bipolar mania or mixed episodes. Olanzapine is approved to treat adolescents aged 13-17 diagnosed with schizophrenia or bipolar disorder (manic or mixed episodes). Off-label prescriptions, however, are often given to younger children for behavioral symptoms, including aggression related to ADHD (Seida et al., 2012); approximately 50% of all antipsychotic medication use is off-label in the American pediatric population (Crystal, Olfson, Huang, Pincus, & Gerhard, 2009).

With regard to European Union countries, aripiprazole was licensed in 2009 by the European Medicine Agency for the treatment of schizophrenia in adolescents aged 15 and older. In several European countries, risperidone is approved for the treatment of children and adolescents with severe disruptive disorders (De Hert, Dobbelaere, Sheridan, Cohen, & Correll, 2011).

CANADIAN SECOND-GENERATION ANTIPSYCHOTIC MEDICATIONS PRESCRIPTION TRENDS FOR CHILDREN AND ADOLESCENTS

At present, the Canadian data on drug prescriptions for youth is limited. In recent years there have been four studies published; three provincial (Manitoba, 2012; Nova Scotia (NS), 2013; and British Columbia (BC), 2013) and one national (2011). The overall trend is similar across the country, with an increase in antipsychotic prescriptions, mainly for SGAs, over time. Notably, the increase in prescriptions cannot be explained by an increase in the youth population, as data from Statistics Canada show that the number of children (persons aged 0-19 years) has slightly decreased each year, from 7,874,686 children in 2005 to 7,863,731 children in 2009. Below, we highlight important prescribing patterns for antipsychotics as reported in the Canadian literature with an emphasis on who is doing the prescribing, what types of antipsychotics are most commonly being prescribed and why, and the characteristics of children and youth who are receiving prescriptions.

NATIONAL PRESCRIBING TRENDS

In 2011, Pringsheim and colleagues (Pringsheim, Lam, & Patten, 2011) performed an analysis of Canadian antipsychotic use by children and youth with the IMS Brogan Canadian CompuScript database and the Canadian Disease and Treatment Index for a 5-year period between 2005 and 2009. They also

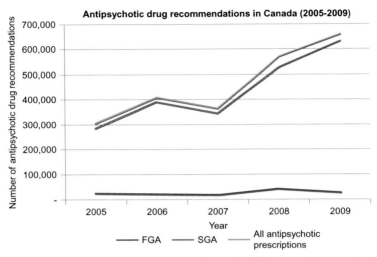

FIGURE 2.1   Yearly antipsychotic drug recommendations for children and adolescents in Canada, 2005-2009.

used IMS Brogan's longitudinal database to estimate the average duration of use of antipsychotics. Their analyses allowed them to analyze drug recommendation frequency and reasons for recommendations (therapeutic indications), as well as duration of use for different types of medications, including antipsychotics, psychostimulants, and selective serotonin reuptake inhibitors (SSRIs). They found that during the 5-year period studied, antipsychotic recommendations for children and adolescents in Canada increased by 114% from 2005 to 2009, from 308,409 drug recommendations in 2005 to 661,300 in 2009 (Figure 2.1).

According to the study, risperidone was the most commonly recommended SGA, followed by quetiapine. Recommendations for both these medications showed an increase on a yearly basis, while recommendations for olanzapine and clozapine remained stable over the same period of time (Figure 2.2). These data suggest that Canadian clinicians are following the literature regarding which medications have been most studied in children with mental disorders, as risperidone has had the greatest number of pediatric trials.

In comparison with the 114% increase in antipsychotic prescriptions, recommendations for psychostimulants over the same time period rose by only 36%, with 1,702,820 recommendations in 2009. Methylphenidate was the most commonly recommended medication. Meanwhile, recommendations for SSRIs increased by 44%, with 518,230 recommendations in 2009 and fluoxetine being the most commonly recommended, followed by citalopram. Thus, it would appear that while prescriptions for psychotropic medications are on the rise overall, antipsychotics represent the fastest-growing class of medications used for the treatment of mental health conditions in children and youth.

The most common reason for an SGA to be prescribed was for a primary diagnosis of ADHD (17%), followed by a mood disorder (16%), conduct disorder

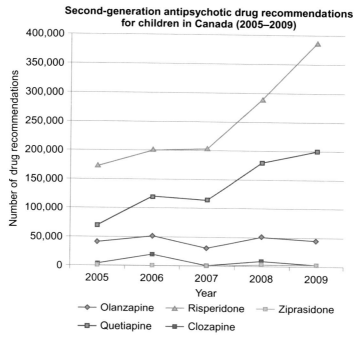

FIGURE 2.2   Yearly second-generation antipsychotic recommendations by medication for children and adolescents in Canada, 2005-2009. Data are not shown for aripiprazole and paliperidone due to overall low numbers.

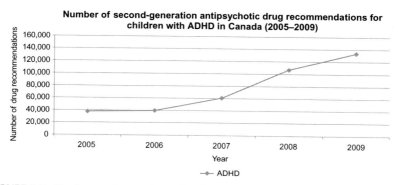

FIGURE 2.3   Yearly second-generation antipsychotic recommendations for children and adolescents with ADHD in Canada, 2005-2009.

(14%), and psychotic disorder (13%). Notably, the number of SGA recommendations for ADHD over the 5-year period more than tripled (Figure 2.3).

Data on the average duration of antipsychotic use by children and adolescents in Canada suggest that these medications are being used for long periods of time. The average duration of antipsychotic use in children varied by drug and age group. For risperidone, the average duration of use was 90 days in children 1-6 years of age, 180 days in children 7-12 years of age, and 200 days in youth 13-18 years of age. Lastly, the Pringsheim study (2011) found that drug recommendations for antipsychotics in young people were made mainly by psychiatrists, with 62% of recommendations, followed by pediatricians and family physicians, each with 17%, and other specialities at just 3%.

PROVINCIAL PRESCRIBING TRENDS

Manitoba

Antipsychotic use in children aged 0-18 years from 1998 to 2008 was studied by Alessi-Severini et al. (2012) using the Manitoba Health Drug Program Information Network database, which collects prescription data for all residents of the province. Their analysis captured 90% of the prescriptions dispensed in the province and provided a comprehensive description of medication use.

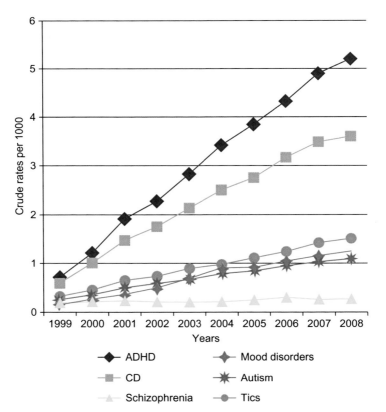

FIGURE 2.4   Diagnoses linked to young antipsychotic users in the province of Manitoba, 1999-2008.

Like the national trend data, the number of prescriptions between 1999 and 2008 increased from 2746 in 1999 to 21,320 in 2008 (Figure 2.4), with more than 96% of prescriptions being for youth aged 7-18. The vast majority of antipsychotics prescribed for children in the province were SGAs (97%). Risperidone was consistently the most common SGA prescribed, with 14,291 prescriptions in 2008, followed by quetiapine with 4636 prescriptions and olanzapine with 2295; these results were consistent with the national trend observed by Pringsheim, Lam, Ching, et al. (2011), Pringsheim, Lam, and Patten (2011), and Pringsheim, Panagiotopoulos, et al. (2011).

In addition to analyzing prescription data, Alessi-Severini et al. (2012) were also able to obtain patient demographic data, including gender, geographic location, and socioeconomic status. Although the study did not identify differences between urban and rural users or between low- and high-income users, they did reveal significant gender-related biases in prescribing patterns. Namely, the number of prescriptions for boys was higher overall and showed an increase from 22.3 per 1000 in 1999 to 103.0 per 1000 in 2008, while prescriptions for girls were more modest, with an increase from 10.8 per 1000 in 1999 to 44.6 per 1000 in 2008. In other words, the male-to-female ratio increased from 1.9:1 in 1999 to 2.3:1 in 2008, with a peak at 2.7:1 in 2005, which is consistent with the higher prevalence of autism and ADHD diagnosed in males.

Accordingly, it was shown that most common reasons for a young person to receive an antipsychotic recommendation in Manitoba was for the treatment of disruptive behavior disorders, ADHD, and conduct disorder. Other diagnoses associated with antipsychotic use were autism, tics, mood disorders, and schizophrenia (Figure 2.4). Unlike the national data, however, the analysis found that in Manitoba, the majority of the prescriptions for SGAs were written by general practitioners (GPs), rather than psychiatrists.

Nova Scotia

Murphy et al. (2013) analyzed prescribing trends of antipsychotics in low-income youth 25 years of age and younger in NS who received drug benefits through the publicly funded Pharmacare program. They used a retrospective population database design to identify the prevalence of antipsychotic prescriptions, type of medication, dose, duration, indication, and prescriber over a 7-year period from 2000 to 2007, through evaluation of antipsychotic prescription claims and health services utilization.

Approximately 4% of Nova Scotians aged 25 and younger (1715 of 43,888 people) who were eligible to receive community service benefits received an antipsychotic prescription between 2000 and 2007. Overall, the study found a significant increase in antipsychotic use in all pediatric age groups, with the exception of young children between 0 and 5 years. Over 30% of all antipsychotic users were 15 years of age or younger. Risperidone

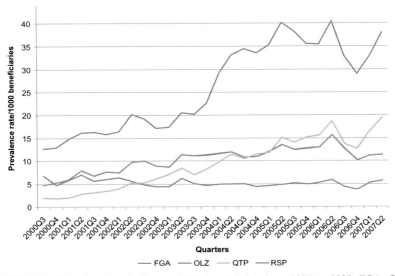

FIGURE 2.5   Use of antipsychotics per 1000 beneficiaries from 2000 to 2007. FGA, first-generation antipsychotic; OLZ, olanzapine; QTP, quetiapine; RSP, risperidone.

was the most common antipsychotic prescribed, followed by quetiapine and olanzapine (Figure 2.5). ADHD was the most attributable diagnosis for risperidone use (31%).

Psychosis was the most common attributable diagnosis when an antipsychotic was initiated (31%), followed by ADHD (16%), anxiety disorders (15%), depression (8%), bipolar disorder (7%), pervasive development disorders (4%), tics (2%), and eating disorders (<1%). Given that psychosis is usually diagnosed in older adolescents and young adults, this finding likely reflects the older age of patients that were included in this study (up to age 25). Interestingly, 66% of those receiving an antipsychotic had two or more psychiatric diagnoses. Thus, it is not surprising that coprescription of antipsychotic medications was also high; 42% of those receiving an antipsychotic were also taking antidepressants, 27% were receiving mood stabilizers, 17% were taking an ADHD medication (stimulants, atomoxetine, or clonidine), and 15% were receiving an anxiolytic. Moreover, the odds of receiving an antipsychotic were 2.5 times greater in males than in females, a finding that echoes the Manitoba data. The median duration of antipsychotic use also varied based on diagnosis and age. The diagnoses associated with the longest use were pervasive developmental disorder and mental retardation, followed by psychotic disorders.

With regard to prescribers, family physicians initiated the majority of the prescriptions (72%), followed by psychiatrists (16%), pediatricians (3%), and others (2%).

British Columbia

A study conducted by Ronsley et al. (2013) used the BC Ministry of Health PharmaNet database to describe antipsychotic prescriptions in children and adolescents aged 18 years and younger. In their analysis, they included antipsychotic type (first- or second-generation), dose, duration of treatment, primary diagnosis, and prescriber by specialty training.

Overall, the prescription of antipsychotics for young people between 1996 and 2011 increased from 1583 in 1996/1997 to 5432 in 2010/2011. This translates into a 3.8-fold increase in the overall antipsychotic prescription use from 1.66 per 1000 in 1996/1997 to 6.37 per 1000 in 2010/2011. Moreover, a shift in favor of SGAs over FGAs was shown over that time period. The total number of youth who received an SGA increased from 315 in 1996/1997 to 5432 in 2010/2011, while the number of prescriptions for FGAs decreased significantly from 1366 to 420 over the same period of time (Figure 2.6). In 1996/1997, 76.3% of antipsychotic prescriptions were for an FGA but by 2010/2011 SGAs accounted for 96% of antipsychotics prescribed in youth.

The most frequently prescribed antipsychotic in BC was risperidone (48%), followed by quetiapine (36%), olanzapine (6%), aripiprazole (3.0%), clozapine (1.4%), ziprasidone (1%), and paliperidone (0.5%).

In concordance with the data from NS and Manitoba, gender-specific biases were also found. For instance, the highest age-specific rate for youth receiving antipsychotic prescriptions was found in males aged 13-18 years, for whom the rate increased from 3.3 per 1000 in 1996/1997 to 14.4 per 1000 in 2010/2011.

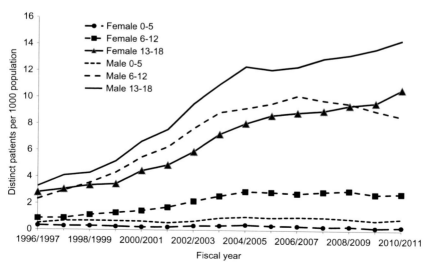

FIGURE 2.6 Yearly trends of antipsychotic prescriptions for children and adolescents in British Columbia, 1996-2011.

Within the same time period, the age-specific rate for females aged 13-18 years increased from 2.8 per 1000 to 10.7 per 1000.

In the BC data set, the three most common diagnoses associated with an antipsychotic prescription were depressive disorders (13%), hyperkinetic syndrome of childhood (12%), and neurotic disorders (11%). However, closer examination of the data revealed differences between age group. In children aged 0-5 years, the most common diagnoses were hyperkinetic syndrome and disturbances of conduct or developmental delay, while in children aged 6-12 years the most common disorder was hyperkinetic syndrome, and in youth aged 13-18 years depression was the most common diagnosis associated with an SGA prescription. Another important finding was that the reasons for prescription varied based on prescriber specialty. GP prescriptions were more commonly linked to a diagnosis of depression or anxiety, while prescriptions made by pediatricians were more often related to behavioral disorders and those made by psychiatrists were due to psychotic disorders. The study also found that the age groups receiving antipsychotics differed depending on prescriber specialty. In 0- to 5-year-olds, the majority of prescriptions were made by pediatricians (47%), followed by family physicians (22%) and psychiatrists (14%). In 6- to 12-year-olds, prescriptions were similar among family physicians, psychiatrists, and pediatricians. In 13- to 18-year-olds, prescriptions were mainly by family physicians and psychiatrists (40% each), with 10% by pediatricians.

COMPARING CANADIAN SGA PRESCRIPTION TRENDS TO THOSE IN OTHER COUNTRIES

According to the scientific literature, there has been a global increase in the use of antipsychotics in children and adolescents and most of that increase can be attributed to SGAs. Our examination of Canadian prescribing trends supports this assertion. However, major differences may still exist regarding the prescription rates and trends for antipsychotics in children and adolescents among different countries (Bachmann, Lempp, Glaeske, & Hoffmann, 2014; De Hert et al., 2011; Patten et al., 2012; Pringsheim, Lam, Ching, et al., 2011; Pringsheim, Lam, & Patten, 2011; Pringsheim, Panagiotopoulos, et al., 2011; Ronsley et al., 2013; Verdoux, Tournier, & Begaud, 2010; Vitiello et al., 2009; Wong, Murray, Camilleri-Novak, & Stephens, 2005; Zito et al., 2008). For instance, the frequency of use of antipsychotics in children and adolescents in Canada appears to be lower than that observed in the United States (Patten et al., 2012). Canadian rates are closer to the estimates of the Netherlands, France, and Iceland and higher than UK and Italian estimates. As reported in a French study, the prevalence of antipsychotic use in those aged 18 and younger in 2004 was 3.4 per 1000, while a study in the Netherlands reported a prevalence of 6.8 per 1000 in those aged 19 and younger in 2005 (Alessi-Severini et al., 2012; Patten et al., 2012).

In a study by Zito et al. (2008), a comparison of the prevalence of psychotropic prescriptions for youth was conducted between the United States, the Netherlands, and Germany. They found that the annual prevalence of any psychotropic medication use by youth was significantly greater in the United States (6.7%) than in the Netherlands (2.9%) and in Germany (2.0%). But among the three countries, Germany had the highest antipsychotic use rate in children aged 0-4 years at 0.64%, followed by the Netherlands (0.10%) and the United States (0.07%). In contrast, the use of other medications by young people, such as stimulants or antidepressants, was three or more times greater in the United States than in the Netherlands and Germany. A recent study by Bachmann et al. (2014) indicates that the rate of antipsychotic prescribing is on the rise in Germany. The percentage of children and adolescents receiving a prescription for an antipsychotic drug rose from 0.23% in 2005 to 0.32% in 2012. This increase was mainly associated with the use of SGAs and was particularly marked in the age group of 10- to 19-year-olds. In these cases, the majority of prescriptions were ordered by either child and adolescent psychiatrists or pediatricians; the most commonly prescribed drugs were risperidone and pipamperone (Bachmann et al., 2014).

CONCLUSIONS

Our review of the prescription rates and trends in Canada and elsewhere has produced many unanswered questions:

1. Why the increase in SGA prescriptions in Canada? According to international literature, there are marked differences between Western Europe and North America in the use of FGAs and SGAs. Currently, U.S. and Canadian data show an almost exclusive use of SGAs in children and adolescents (Patten et al., 2012). In contrast, the use of FGAs is still quite prevalent in Europe, although a significant shift toward more frequent use of SGAs has been reported.

2. What factors other than disease prevalence contribute to our gender-specific findings? According to Zito et al. (2008), rates of antipsychotic use are also significantly higher for males. However, it has been shown that the male-to-female ratio is lower in Germany (1.4:1) compared to the Netherlands (3.2:1) and the United States (2.8:1). In the Canadian studies we reviewed above, the male/female ratios were most similar to those observed in the United States (2.3:1).

3. What role does culture play, if any, in determining whether or not an antipsychotic is recommended? In some countries, such as Australia, the use of SGAs in children and youth has remained relatively stable (Hollingsworth, Duhig, Hall, & Scott, 2013). Why is this the case? Some of the differences in prescribing patterns might be explained by sociocultural factors, as these influence attitudes toward mental disorders in children and adolescents as well as the utilization of psychotropics for young people. Differences can also be

explained by variation in the structure of and access to health services, drug regulation, and the diagnostic system utilized. Other factors that may be related to changes in SGA prescription for children include the level of awareness regarding mental disorders, underreporting of negative side effects by health providers, and adherence to evidence-based clinical guidelines by health care providers (Vitiello et al., 2009). In some countries, aggressive drug company advertising, including marketing to doctors and direct-to-consumer advertising, plays an important role. According to various studies, the use of SGAs for a longer duration might explain the increased rate of use (Patten et al., 2012; Pringsheim, Lam, Ching, et al., 2011; Pringsheim, Lam, & Patten, 2011; Pringsheim, Panagiotopoulos, et al., 2011). Further studies are needed to elucidate these questions and the reasons for the growing use of antipsychotics.

Canada, like other developed countries, has seen a large increase in antipsychotic medication prescribing for youth for a variety of mental health conditions over the past decade. Strategies to promote the safe and rational use of antipsychotic medications in children are important to the education of physicians and parents regarding the role of antipsychotics in the management of childhood mental health disorders and the need for safety monitoring.

REFERENCES

Alessi-Severini, S., Biscontri, R., Collins, D., Sareen, J., & Enns, M. (2012). Ten years of antipsychotic prescribing to children: A Canadian population-based study. *Canadian Journal of Psychiatry, 57*(1), 52–58.

Bachmann, C., Lempp, T., Glaeske, G., & Hoffmann, F. (2014). Antipsychotic prescription in children and adolescents: An analysis of data from a German statutory health insurance company from 2005 to 2012. *Deutsches Ärzteblatt International, 111*(3), 25–34.

Canada Adverse Reaction Newsletter. (2012). (Vol. 22). Health Canada.

Cooper, W., Arbogast, P., & Ding, H. (2006). Trends in prescribing of antipsychotic medications for US children. *Ambulatory Pediatrics, 6*, 79–83.

Crystal, S., Olfson, M., Huang, C., Pincus, H., & Gerhard, T. (2009). Broadened use of atypical antipsychotics: Safety, effectiveness, and policy challenges. *Health Affairs (Millwood), 28*(5), w770–w781.

De Hert, M., Dobbelaere, M., Sheridan, E., Cohen, D., & Correll, C. (2011). Metabolic and endocrine adverse effects of second-generation antipsychotics in children and adolescents: A systematic review of randomized, placebo controlled trials and guidelines for clinical practice. *European Psychiatry, 26*(3), 144–158.

Doey, T., Handelman, K., & Seabrook, J. (2007). Survey of atypical antipsychotic prescribing by Canadian child psychiatrists and developmental pediatricians for patients aged under 18 years. *Canadian Journal of Psychiatry, 52*, 363–368.

Gardner, D. M., & Teehan, M. D. (2010). *The antipsychotics and their side effects*. Cambridge, UK: Cambridge University Press.

Hollingsworth, S., Duhig, M., Hall, W., & Scott, J. (2013). National trends in the community prescribing of second-generation antipsychotic medications in Australian children and youth: The incomplete story. *Australasian Psychiatry, 21*(5), 442–445.

Luo, X., Doherty, J., Cappelleri, J., & Frush, K. (2007). Role of pharmacoepidemiology in evaluating prescription drug safety in pediatrics. *Current Medical Research and Opinion, 23*(11), 2607–2615.

Morrato, E., Nicol, G., & Maahs, D. (2010). Metabolic screening in children receiving antipsychotic drug treatment. *Archives of Pediatrics and Adolescent Medicine, 164*, 344–351.

Murphy, A., Gardner, D. M., Cooke, C., Kisely, S., Hughes, J., & Kutcher, S. (2013). Prescribing trends of antipsychotics in youth receiving income assistance: Results from a retrospective population database study. *BMC Psychiatry, 13*(1), 198.

Patel, N., Crismon, M., Hoagwood, K., Johnsrud, M., Rascati, K., Wilson, J., et al. (2005). Trends in the use of typical and atypical antipsychotics in children and adolescents. *Journal of the American Academy of Child and Adolescent Psychiatry, 44*(6), 548–556.

Patten, S., Waheed, W., & Bresee, L. (2012). A review of pharmacoepidemiologic studies of antipsychotic use in children and adolescents. *Canadian Journal of Psychiatry, 57*(12), 717–721.

Pierre, J. (2005). Extrapyramidal symptoms with atypical antipsychotics: Incidence, prevention and management. *Drug Safety, 28*(3), 191–208.

Prince, M., Patel, V., Saxena, S., Maj, M., Maselko, J., Phillips, M., et al. (2007). No health without mental health. *Lancet, 370*(9590), 859–877.

Pringsheim, T., Lam, D., Ching, H., & Patten, S. (2011). Metabolic and neurological complications of second-generation antipsychotic use in children: A systematic review and meta-analysis of randomized controlled trials. *Drug Safety, 34*(8), 651–668.

Pringsheim, T., Lam, D., & Patten, S. (2011). The pharmacoepidemiology of antipsychotic medications for Canadian children and adolescents: 2005–2009. *Journal of Child and Adolescent Psychopharmacology, 21*(6), 536–543.

Pringsheim, T., Panagiotopoulos, C., Davidson, J., Ho, J., The Canadian Alliance for Monitoring Effectiveness and Safety of Antipsychotics in Children (CAMESA) guideline group. (2011). Evidence-based recommendations for monitoring safety of second-generation antipsychotics in children and youth. *Paediatrics and Child Health, 16*(9), 581–589.

Ronsley, R., Scott, D., Warburton, W., Hamdi, R., Louie, D., Davidson, J., et al. (2013). A population-based study of antipsychotic prescription trends in children and adolescents in British Columbia, from 1996 to 2011. *Canadian Journal of Psychiatry, 58*(6), 361–369.

Seida, J., Schouten, J., Mousavi, S., Hamm, M., Beaith, A., Vandermeer, B., et al. (2012). First- and second-generation antipsychotics for children and young adults (Internet).

Verdoux, H., Tournier, M., & Begaud, B. (2010). Antipsychotic prescribing trends: A review of pharmaco-epidemiological studies. *Acta Psychiatrica Scandinavica, 121*(1), 4–10.

Vitiello, B., Correll, C., van Zwiten-Boot, B., Zuddas, A., Parallada, M., & Arango, C. (2009). Antipsychotics in children and adolescents: Increasing use, evidence for efficacy and safety concerns. *European Neuropsychopharmacology, 19*(9), 629–635.

Wong, I., Murray, M., Camilleri-Novak, D., & Stephens, P. (2005). Increased prescribing trends of paediatric psychotropic medications. *Archives of Disease in Childhood, 89*(12), 1131–1132.

World Health Organization, WHO International Working Group for Drug Statistics Methodology, WHO Collaborating Centre for Drug Statistics Methodology, & WHO Collaborating Centre for Drug Utilization Research and Clinical Pharmacological Services. (2003). *Introduction to drug utilization research.* Oslo, Norway: WHO Press.

Zito, J., Safer, D., de Jong-van den Berg, L., Janhsen, K., Fegert, J., Gardner, J., et al. (2008). A three-country comparison of psychotropic medication prevalence in youth. *Child and Adolescent Psychiatry and Mental Health, 2*(1), 26.

Chapter 3

Do We Know If They Work and If They Are Safe: Second-Generation Antipsychotics for Treatment of Autism Spectrum Disorders and Disruptive Behavior Disorders in Children and Adolescents

Dean Elbe[*,†], Edel Mc Glanaghy[‡], Tim F. Oberlander[§]

[*]*Division of Children's and Women's Mental Health, BC Mental Health & Addiction Services, Vancouver, British Columbia, Canada*

[†]*Department of Pharmacy, BC Children's Hospital, Vancouver, British Columbia, Canada*

[‡]*National Core for Neuroethics, Division of Neurology, Faculty of Medicine, University of British Columbia, Vancouver, British Columbia, Canada*

[§]*Department of Pediatrics, School of Population and Public Health, University of British Columbia, Vancouver, British Columbia, Canada*

INTRODUCTION

Over the past 20 years, large increases in usage rates of second-generation antipsychotics (SGAs; for the purposes of this chapter also includes aripiprazole, technically a third-generation antipsychotic) by children and adolescents have been observed, with reported increases ranging from 4- to 18-fold over this time period (Alessi-Severini, Biscontri, Collins, Sareen, & Enns, 2012; Harrison, Cluxton-Keller, & Gross, 2012; Olfson, He, & Merikangas, 2013; Ronsley et al., 2013; Therapeutics Initiative, 2009). Such rapid expansion of SGA prescribing has been met with significant concern on the part of parents and caregivers, physicians and healthcare professionals, and both professional and lay media (Belluz, 2012; Chance, 2013; Jacobson, 2014; Kirkey, 2013; Reinberg, 2012; Vitiello et al., 2009).

As of September 2014, aripiprazole is the only SGA that has Health Canada approval for use in children age 15 and up for treatment of schizophrenia and age 13 and up for treatment of bipolar mania. None of the other available SGAs (asenapine (Saphris®), clozapine (Clozaril®), lurasidone (Latuda®), olanzapine (Zyprexa®), paliperidone (Invega®), quetiapine (Seroquel®), risperidone (Risperdal®), or ziprasidone (Zeldox®) are currently approved by Health Canada for any indication in pediatric patients. Other than for aripiprazole as described above, SGAs, when prescribed for treatment of children and adolescents in Canada, are used on an "off-label" basis.

A lack of regulatory approval by Health Canada however does not automatically mean there is no evidence to support the use of SGAs for treatment of autism spectrum disorders (ASDs) and disruptive behavior disorders (DBDs) in the pediatric population. The body of pediatric psychopharmacology research has increased dramatically during the last 15 years, partly due to U.S. incentivizing legislation. The Best Pharmaceuticals for Children Act (BPCA: U.S. Food and Drug Administration, 2002). passed by the U.S. federal government in 2002 provided incentives to pharmaceutical companies to conduct pediatric medication trials. This legislation has had an impact reaching well beyond the U.S. borders. The BPCA granted pharmaceutical companies an additional 6 months of U.S. market patent protection for all dosage forms, indications, and age groups following completion of at least one randomized controlled trial (RCT) in the pediatric population. Antipsychotic medications such as aripiprazole (and risperidone, olanzapine, and quetiapine prior to their patent expiry dates) are top-selling drugs in the United States annually. An extra 6 months of patent protection and U.S. market exclusivity for an SGA can be worth upward of $2 billion in extra revenue to a company.

Use of SGAs in children and adolescents is relatively well studied and accepted for the treatment of schizophrenia and bipolar mania, and U.S. Food and Drug Administration (FDA) approval has been granted for several of the SGAs for these indications. Dramatic increases in office visits in the past two decades (Moreno et al., 2007) pertaining to the diagnosis of pediatric bipolar disorder alongside an observed increase in pediatric SGA utilization rates have generated a large amount of controversy surrounding pediatric bipolar disorder as a valid diagnosis, particularly as the behavioral presentation for pediatric bipolar disorder may be similar to that of other childhood behavior disorders (Tusaie, 2010). Subsequently, pediatric bipolar disorder has recently been re-conceptualized in the Diagnostic and Statistical Manual of Mental Disorders, 5th Edition (DSM-5: APA, 2013), as disruptive mood dysregulation disorder (DMDD), a mood disorder in children characterized by frequent irritable moods, but outside the bipolar spectrum.

This diagnostic confusion has led to a situation where the literature may be misunderstood and useful information about the benefits of SGAs in children may have been overlooked. While it is hoped that this recent change in the DSM-5 may lead to more clarity around childhood bipolar disorder by allowing more consistent study categories and thereby assisting our understanding about who might best benefit from SGA treatment, it is prudent to consider studies that took place prior to DSM-5 that involve pediatric bipolar disorder as they may be relevant to the DBD literature.

For this chapter, we chose to examine in detail two of the more controversial uses for SGAs in pediatric patients: treatment of irritability associated with ASDs and treatment of DBDs. Often, but not always, DBDs encompass patients with attention-deficit/hyperactivity disorder (ADHD), which in DSM-5 is a diagnosis under the broader category of DBDs. Both ASDs and DBDs are conditions that may be marked by the presence of the nonspecific symptom of aggression, which has sometimes been called "the fever of child psychiatry."

Medication nomenclature issues also may contribute to the angst and confusion surrounding the antipsychotic medication category. There is no marketed category of anti-aggressive medications. Drugs which act to reduce dopamine activity and increase serotonin activity appear to be effective for treatment of impulsive aggression, and this profile most closely resembles the primary pharmacological actions of SGAs (Swann, 2003). However, medication category names are assigned (and retained) based on their historical first approved indication, which in the case of antipsychotic drugs was for treatment of schizophrenia (psychosis) (King & Voruganti, 2002). While the FDA has approved aripiprazole and risperidone for treatment of irritability associated with ASDs (Janssen Pharmaceuticals Inc., 2013; Otsuka Pharmaceutical Co. Abilify (aripiprazole), 2013), no SGAs are FDA approved for treatment of DBDs. At present, Health Canada has not approved any medication for treatment of ASDs or DBDs.

METHODS

We performed two systematic literature searches using the same methodology. Four databases were used; Medline, EMbase, Central (using Ovid), and Psychinfo (using EBSCOhost), with search dates of January 1, 1990 to September 9, 2014. Search terms included Cochrane filters for clinical trials (where available), the nine SGA medications available in Canada (aripiprazole, asenapine, clozapine, lurasidone, olanzapine, paliperidone, quetiapine, risperidone, and ziprasidone) and one of the following.

- ASD: Children and adolescents up to and including age 18 years only with a diagnosis of autism, autistic disorder, ASD, Asperger syndrome, pervasive developmental disorder, or pervasive developmental disorder, not otherwise specified. The DSM-5, released in 2013, combined all of these conditions under the diagnosis of ASD but historical terms for these disorders were used to ensure all relevant literature was identified.
- DBD: Children and adolescents up to and including age 18 years only with a diagnosis of a DBD, including but not limited to conduct disorder (CD), oppositional defiant disorder (ODD), ADHD, DBD not otherwise specified, or aggressive behavior.

After duplicate search results were removed, one author reviewed the titles and abstracts of all the articles obtained through the search strategy and excluded those that were not relevant. The full text of the remaining articles was retrieved and considered against the full inclusion criteria. Eight RCTs remained from the ASD search, and nine from the DBD search. See Figures 3.1 and 3.2 for full details.

Upon examination of the full text, articles were excluded for the following reasons: not report of clinical trial data (14% in ASD search and 28% in DBD search), trial did not have an RCT design (38% and 35%, respectively), trial did not include one of the nine SGAs or placebo (21% in ASD and 30% in DBD), and trial involved either a post hoc analysis, a drug discontinuation design, or measured the impact of an adjunct treatment rather than the antipsychotic (26% and 7%, respectively).

Information about each RCT was extracted and tabulated, including the study design, participant details, intervention, outcome results, and safety data. The trial data are presented in Tables 3.1 and 3.2 and summarized below. A full list of the trial references is presented at the end of the reference

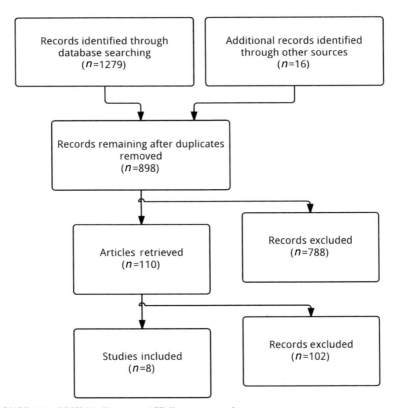

FIGURE 3.1   PRISMA diagram—ASD literature search.

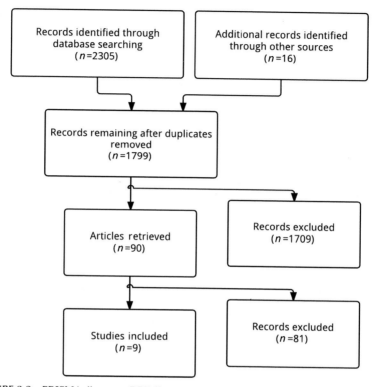

FIGURE 3.2   PRISMA diagram—DBD literature search.

section. A concise summary of the most commonly used outcome measures can be found in Box 3.1, with side effect measures in Box 3.2.

Efficacy of SGAs for Children and Adolescents With ASDs

Eight RCTs which compared SGAs to placebo for irritability/behavioral issues associated with ASDs were identified: two with aripiprazole, one with olanzapine, and five with risperidone. No RCTs for treatment of ASDs were identified for asenapine, clozapine, lurasidone, quetiapine, paliperidone, or ziprasidone. A summary of these RCTs can be found in Table 3.1. All but two trials provided dates for when the trials took place. These were conducted between 1999 and 2010 and all trials were published between 2002 and 2013. Six trials were conducted in the United States, one in Canada and one in India. The number of treatment sites per trial ranged between 1 and 37 sites, and in 6 of the 8 trials funding for the study was provided by the pharmaceutical company that manufactured the SGA studied.

The trials ranged in size from 11 to 218 participants, with a total of 667 children enrolled. Most RCTs applied an intention to treat (ITT) analysis (an approach used to provide unbiased comparisons among the treatment groups).

TABLE 3.1 Published Randomized Controlled Trials of SGAs for ASDs in Children and Adolescents

Lead Author, Year, Journal	n, % ♂, Age (Years) Range, Mean Age (sd)	Drug/Dose; Duration	Concurrent Medications	Primary Outcome#	Secondary Outcomes	Weight Change/ Metabolic Effects	Adverse Effects
Aripiprazole							
Marcus et al. (2009); *J Am Acad Child Adolesc Psychiatry*	n=218 90% ♂; Age range 6-17 PBO: 10.2±3.1 A5: 9±2.8 A10: 10±3.2 A15: 9.5±3.1	Fixed dose: 5 mg/day, 10 mg/day, or 15 mg/day 8-week duration	Analgesics/ antipyretics 21%, anticholinergics 4%, anxiolytics 3%, hypnotics/ sedatives 3%, propranolol 1%	ABC-irritability A5: −12.4** A10: −13.2** A15: −14.4** PBO: −8.4 CGI-I A5: 2.6** A10: 2.5** A15: 2.5** PBO: 3.3	*Statistically significant results* ABC-hyperactivity ABC-stereotypy ABC-inappropriate speech (A15mg only) CGI-S (A10mg, 15 mg only) Response: ABC-I score ≥25% improvement plus CGI-I ≤2 (A5 only) cY-BOCS (A15 only) CGI-S score (A10, A15 only) PedsQL (A15 only) CGSQ (A15 only) *Nonsignificant results* ABC-social withdrawal/lethargy	*Weight change* A5: +1.3±0.3 kg** A10: +1.3±0.3 kg** A15: +1.5±0.3 kg** PBO: +0.3±0.3 kg *BMI change* A5: +0.6±0.2 kg/m² A10: +0.6±0.2 kg/m² A15: +0.8±0.2 kg/m²** PBO: +0.2±0.2 kg/m² *Prolactin change* A5: −5.4 ng/ml** A10: −5.2 ng/ml**	##*Neurological* EPS 4-11%, tremor 8-12%, somnolence 4-5%, fatigue 4-22%, headache 2-5%, lethargy 5-8%, pyrexia/ fever 6-12%, sedation 11-23%, hypersomnia 0-6% *HEENT* thirst 0-4%, drooling 4-14%, hypersalivation 0-9% *Respiratory* URTI 0-6%, nasopharyngitis 5-8%, nasal congestion 0-5%, epistaxis 0-7%, rhinorrhea 0-7%, cough-4-11% *Gastrointestinal* abdominal pain 0-5%, increased appetite 1-15%, vomiting 2-12%, nausea 0-5%, decreased appetite 4-7%, weight gain 0-6%, gastroenteritis 2-5%

| Owen et al. (2009); *Pediatrics* | $n=98$ 88% ♂; Age range 6-17 A: 9.7±3.2 PBO: 8.8±2.6 | Flexible dose Mean 8.9 mg/day, Range 2-15 mg/day 8 weeks duration | Any medication 36%: analgesic/antipyretic 21%, hypnotic/sedatives 7%, benztropine 1% | ABC-irritability A: −12.9** PBO: −5 (ES 0.87) CGI-I ≤2 A: 67%** PBO: 16% | *Statistically significant results* ABC-hyperactivity ABC-stereotypy ABC-inappropriate speech CGI-S Response: ABC-I ≥25% plus CGI-I ≤2 cY-BOCS *Nonsignificant results* ABC-social withdrawal/lethargy PedsQL CGSQ | *Weight change* A: +1.9 kg** PBO: +0.5 kg- make sure matches text *BMI change* A: +0.7 kg/m² PBO: +0.3 kg/m² *Prolactin change* A: −6.3 ng/ml** PBO: +1.6 ng/ml No significant difference in FBG, TG, LDL, HDL, Tchol | Any adverse effect 20% *Neurological* fatigue 17%, somnolence 13%, tremor 9%, sedation 9%, pyrexia/fever 7%, extrapyramidal disorder 2%, hypokinesia 2%, rigidity 1% *HEENT* drooling 9% *Respiratory* nasal congestion 4% *Gastrointestinal* vomiting 11%, increased appetite 5% Notes on SAE: A ($n=1$) "mild intensity" suicide related behavior AE "not related to treatment" PBO ($n=3$) "moderate intensity" suicide related behavior, "probably related to treatment" |
| | | | | | A15: −5.8 ng/ml** PBO: +0.9 ng/ml No significant differences in FBG, TG, LDL, HDL, TChol | *Genitourinary* enuresis (−2)-4% *Dermatological* rash (−2)-3% |

Continued

TABLE 3.1 Published Randomized Controlled Trials of SGAs for ASDs in Children and Adolescents—Cont'd

Lead Author, Year; Journal	n, % ♂, Age (Years) Range, Mean Age (sd)	Drug/Dose; Duration	Concurrent Medications	Primary Outcome#	Secondary Outcomes	Weight Change/ Metabolic Effects	Adverse Effects
Olanzapine							
Hollander et al. (2006); *J Child Adolesc Psychopharmacol*	n=11 82% ♂; Age range 6-14	Flexible dose§ (<40 kg, ≥40 kg) "Overall" mean 10±2.04 mg/ day	No information provided	CGI-I O: −1.75 PBO: −0.5	Nonsignificant results cY-BOCS compulsion subscale	Weight change O: +3.4±2.2 kg**	Neurological sedation 47%, insomnia 17% HEENT glazed eyes 17%
	O: 9.25±2.9 PBO: 8.9±2.1	Range 7.5-12.5 mg/day 8-week duration		"Responders" (measure not specified) O: 50% PBO: 20%	OAS-M irritability and aggression subscales	PBO: +0.7±0.7 kg	Respiratory rhinitis 17% Gastrointestinal constipation 50% increased appetite 10%, decreased appetite 17%, mild weight gain 33%, severe weight gain 33% No SAE
Risperidone							
Kent et al. (2013); *J Autism Dev Disord*	n=96 88% ♂; Age range 5-17 R low dose: 10±3.4 R high dose: 9±3.1 PBO: 9±2.6	Fixed dose§ R low dose 20-45 kg: 0.125 mg/day ≥45 kg 0.175 mg/day R high dose 20-45 kg: 1.25 mg/day	Antihistamines 10%	ABC-irritability R low dose: −7.4 R high dose: −12.4** PBO: −3.5 ES: R low dose 0.36,	Statistically significant results Response rate: improved at least 25% on ABC-irritability (R high dose only) CGI-I % <3(R high dose only)	Weight change R low dose: +1.2±1.1 kg R high dose: +2.4±2.1 kg PBO: +0.7±1.2 kg BMI change R low dose: +0.4±0.7 kg/m²	Any adverse effect (−20)-7% Neurological sedation 3-26% somnolence (−3)-20%, depression 0-6%, akathisia (−3)-3%, pyrexia/fever 0-6%, hypersomnia (−3)-3% HEENT thirst 0-6%

Do We Know If They Work and If They Are Safe

		≥45 kg 1.75 mg/day 6-week duration	R high dose 0.94	ABC-hyperactivity (R high dose only) ABC-stereotypy (R low dose only) CGI-S (R high dose only) cY-BOCS compulsion scale (R high dose only) *Nonsignificant results* ABC-social withdrawal/lethargy ABC-inappropriate speech	R high dose: +1.1 ± 1.4 kg/m² PBO: +0.1 ± 0.7 kg/m² *Prolactin change* R low dose: +2.58 ng/ml R high dose: +20.23 ng/ml PBO: +1.27 ng/ml No significant differences in FBG, TG, TChol, LDL, HDL.	*Respiratory* URTI 0-7%, nasopharyngitis 1-7%, epistaxis 0-6%, ear infection 0-6% *Gastrointestinal* increased appetite 11-29%, weight gain 4-7%, abdominal pain 3-6%, constipation (−3)-3%, vomiting 0-1%, nausea 0-3% *Genitourinary* enuresis 6-7% *Dermatological* rash 0-7% SAE notes: Oligomenorrhea present in 3% R high dose group
Luby et al. (2006); *J Child Adolesc Psycho-pharmacol*	n = 24 74% ♂; Age range 2.5-6 R: 4.1 ± 0.9 PBO: 4 ± 1.1	Flexible-dose: Mean 1.14 ± 0.32 mg/day, 0.05 mg/kg/day Range 0.50-1.5 mg/day 26-week duration	*No information provided*	CARS R: −4.6** PBO: −1.8 GARS "no significant time by treatment interaction" *Nonsignificant results* VABS CBCL	*Weight change* R: +2.96 ± 2.5 kg** PBO: +0.6 ± 1.1 kg *Prolactin change* R: +33.4 ± 14.5 ng/ ml** PBO: +11.1 ± 18.7 ng/ml No significant difference in leptin levels	*Neurological* sedation 12%, staring spells 9% *HEENT* hypersalivation 18% *Gastrointestinal* increased appetite 30%, constipation 9%

Continued

TABLE 3.1 Published Randomized Controlled Trials of SGAs for ASDs in Children and Adolescents—Cont'd

Lead Author, Year; Journal	n, % ♂, Age (Years) Range, Mean Age (sd)	Drug/Dose; Duration	Concurrent Medications	Primary Outcome#	Secondary Outcomes	Weight Change/ Metabolic Effects	Adverse Effects
RUPPAN (2002); N Engl J Med	n = 101 81% ♂; Age range 5-17 Mean 8.8 ± 2.7	Flexible dose§ (<20 kg, 20-45 kg, >45 kg) Mean 1.8 ± 0.7 mg/day Range 0.5-3.5 mg/day 8-week duration	Anticon-vulsants 4%	ABC-Irritability R: −14.9** (ES 1.2) PBO: −3.6 Response: ABC-I ≥ 25% improvement plus CGI-I ≤2) R: 69%** PBO: 12%	*Statistically significant results* ABC-hyperactivity ABC-stereotypy ABC-social withdrawal/lethargy ABC-inappropriate Speech CGI-I (% improved)	*Weight change* R: +2.7 ± 2.9 kg** PBO: +0.8 ± 2.2 kg No significant difference in pulse, BP, lab tests	*Neurological* drowsiness 37%, fatigue 32%, tremor 12%, dizziness 12%, muscle rigidity 8%, dyskinesia 6%, headache 6%, difficulty sleeping 4%, anxiety 4% *HEENT* drooling 21%, dry mouth 8%, thirst 2% *Cardiovascular* tachycardia 10% *Respiratory* nasal congestion 12%, sore throat 8%, URTI 6% *Gastrointestinal* increased appetite 44%, constipation 17%, vomiting 9% *Genitourinary* enuresis 2% *Dermatological* skin irritation 8% No SAE

				CARS / ABC measure	Statistically significant results	Weight change	Adverse effects
Nagaraj et al. (2006); *J Child Neurol*	n=40 87% ♂; Age range 2-9 R: 4.83±1.74 PBO: 5.25±1.68	Fixed dose 1 mg/day 26-week duration	Antiepileptic drugs allowed	CARS median score/% improved by ≥20% R: −7.5** 63%** PBO: −1 0% CGAS mean/% with ≥20% score increase R: 11.15** 89%** PBO: 2.55 10%	*Statistically significant results* 17-item measure: responsiveness, nonverbal communication, decreased symptoms hyperactivity scales *Nonsignificant results* Global Impression of Parents *Restricted issues, emotional interactions, verbal communication or speech*	*Weight change* R: +2.8±2.0kg PBO: +1.7±1.3 kg	*Neurological* sedation 21%^, dyskinesia 16%^ *HEENT* drooling 5%^ *Gastrointestinal* increased appetite and improved eating habits 89%^
Shea et al. (2004); *Pediatrics*	n=79 79% ♂; Age range 5-12 R: 7.6±2.3 PBO: 7.3±2.3	Flexible dose Mean 1.48mg/ day, 0.05mg/kg/day Range: 0.02-0.06mg/kg/day 8-week duration	Any 79% analgesics 28%, cough & cold preparations 18%, antibiotics 13%, anti-asthmatics 13%, hypnotics/sedatives 25%, anticholinergics 5%	ABC-irritability R: −31** PBO: −27.7	*Statistically significant results* ABC-hyperactivity ABC-stereotypy ABC-social withdrawal/lethargy ABC-inappropriate speech NCBRF VAS (most troublesome symptoms) CGI-C (equivalent to CGI-I)	*Weight change* R: +2.7±2.0kg** PBO: +1.0±1.6kg *Pulse rate change* R: +8.9± 13.9bpm** PBO: −0.6±13.1 bpm *SBP change* R: +4.0± 10.4mmHg** PBO: −0.7±10.7 mmHg Clinically important electrocardiogram changes	Any adverse effect 20% *Neurological* somnolence 65%, apathy 13%, tremor 10%, headache 8%, fatigue 7%, extrapyramidal disorder 5%^, hypokinesis 5%^, influenza-like symptoms 5%, pyrexia 2% *HEENT* hypersalivation 7% *Cardiovascular* tachycardia 13% *Respiratory* URTI 23%, rhinitis 18%, cough 5%

Continued

TABLE 3.1 Published Randomized Controlled Trials of SGAs for ASDs in Children and Adolescents—Cont'd

Lead Author, Year, Journal	n, % δ, Age (Years) Range, Mean Age (sd)	Drug/Dose; Duration	Concurrent Medications	Primary Outcome#	Secondary Outcomes	Weight Change/ Metabolic Effects	Adverse Effects
						R: 3% No significant ESRS differences	*Gastrointestinal* increased appetite 13%, abdominal pain 12%, constipation 10%, weight gain 7%, anorexia 7% SAE: R (n=5): 1 hyperkinesia/somnolence, 1 weight gain, somnolence, 1 aggressive reaction/impaired concentration, 1 extrapyramidal disorder PBO (n=2): 1 insomnia & sunken eyes, 1 accidental medication overdose

Abbreviations: A=aripiprazole; A5=aripiprazole 5 mg; A10=aripiprazole 10 mg; A15=aripiprazole 15 mg; BMI=body mass index; EPS=extrapyramidal symptoms; ES=effect size; FBG=fasting blood glucose; HDL=high-density lipoprotein; HEENT=head, eyes, ears, nose, and throat; LDL=low-density lipoprotein; MPH=methylphenidate; N/A=not available; O=olanzapine; PBO=placebo; R=risperidone; SAE=serious adverse event; SBP: systolic blood pressure; Tchol=total cholesterol; TG=triglycerides; URTI=upper respiratory tract infection; δ=male; †=positive score denotes improvement; ∧=% in treatment group, no information on placebo group; **=statistically significant result; §=weight consideration for dosage; #=primary outcome scores refer to "mean change from baseline."

Abbreviations of rating scales used: ABC: Aberrant Behavior Checklist; ABC-I: Aberrant Behavior Checklist (Irritability subscale); CARS: Childhood Autism Rating Scale; CBCL: Child Behavior Checklist; CGI-C: Clinical Global Impression-Change (equivalent of CGI-I); CGI-I: Clinical Global Impression-Improvement; CGI-S: Clinical Global Impression-Severity; CGAS: Children's Global Assessment Scale; CGSQ: Caregiver Strain Questionnaire; cY-BOCS: Children's Yale-Brown Obsessive-Compulsive Scale; ESRS: Extrapyramidal Symptom Rating Scale; GARS: Gilliam Autism Rating Scale; NCBRF: Nisonger Child Behavior Rating Form; OAS-M: Overt Aggression Scale-Modified; PedsQL: Pediatric Quality of Life Inventory; VABS: Vineland Adaptive Behavior Scale; VAS: Visual Analog Scale.

Note: ## The adverse effects for A5 mg, A10 mg, and A15 mg are presented as a range; however, the upper end of the range was mainly associated with the A10-mg dose.

TABLE 3.2 Published Randomized Controlled Trials of SGAs for DBDs in Children and Adolescents

Lead Author, Year, Journal	n; % ♂; Age (Years): Range, Mean Age	Drug/Dose; Duration	Concurrent Medications	Primary Outcome#	Secondary Outcomes	Weight Change/ Metabolic Effects	Adverse Effects
Aripiprazole							
Tramontina et al. (2009); J Clin Psychiatry	n = 43 47% ♂; Age range 8-17 A: 11.72 ± 2.71 PBO: 12.16 ± 2.75	Flexible dose§ (<50kg, ≥50kg) Mean 13.61 ± 5.37 mg/day Range 5-20mg/ day 6-week duration	None	YMRS A: −27.22** PBO: −19.52 ES 0.80 SNAP-IV A: 0.79 PBO: 0.55	Statistically significant results CMRS CGI-S Nonsignificant results CDRS-R KADS	Weight change A: +1.2 kg PBO: +0.7 kg BMI change No significant change No significant change in "lab tests"	Neurological tiredness 26%, somnolence 21%, neck rigidity 17%, headache 16%, tremor 15%, hostility 14%, sweating 14%, confusion 11%, EPS 11%, blurred vision 8%, change in reflexes 6%, fever/pyrexia 6%, suicidal ideation 6%, oculogyric crisis 6%, itches 5%, dizziness 4%, memory impairment 2%, photosensitivity 2%, HEENT sialorrhea 17% Respiratory breathless 5%, cough 4%, chest pain 1% Gastrointestinal vomiting 17%, nausea 15%, decreased appetite 11% Dermatological edema 13%, dry skin 1%

Continued

TABLE 3.2 Published Randomized Controlled Trials of SGAs for DBDs in Children and Adolescents—Cont'd

Lead Author, Year, Journal	n; % δ; Age (Years): Range, Mean Age	Drug/Dose; Duration	Concurrent Medications	Primary Outcome#	Secondary Outcomes	Weight Change/ Metabolic Effects	Adverse Effects
Quetiapine							
Connor et al. (2008); J Child Adolesc Psychopharmacol	n=19 74% δ Age range 12-17 Q: 13.1±1.2 PBO: 15±1.4	Flexible-dose Mean 294±78mg/day Range 200-600mg/day 7-week duration	None	CGI-S Q: −2.5** PBO:−0.5 CGI-I ≤2 at endpoint Q: 89%** PBO: 10%	Statistically significant results Q-LES-Q Nonsignificant results OAS total CPRS	Weight change Q: +2.3 kg PBO: +1.1 kg BMI change No difference across groups Prolactin change Q: +7.1±2.7 ng/ml PBO: +7.6±4.7 ng/ ml Q: higher average sitting pulse rate) No difference ECGs or QRS, lab measures and no neurological side effects	Neurological restlessness 8% HEENT drooling 22% Gastrointestinal weight gain 23%

Risperidone

Aman et al. (2002); Am J Psychiatry	Flexible dose	No information provided	NCBRF-conduct	Statistically significant results	Weight change	Any 28%
n=118	Mean		R: −15.2**	NCBRF-competent	R: +2.2 ± 1.8 kg**	*Neurological* somnolence 41%,
82% ♂;	1.16±0.57 mg/		PBO: −6.2	calm	PBO: +0.9 ± 1.5 kg	headache 15%, elevated serum
Age range	day, 0.04 mg/			NCBRF-adaptive/social	*Prolactin change*	prolactin 11%, rhinitis 6%,
5-12	kg/day			NCBRF-insecure/	R: +30.7 ng/ml	EPS 4%^
R: 8.7 ±2.1	Range 0.006-			anxious	PBO: +2.5 ng/ml	*Gastrointestinal* vomiting 14%,
PBO:	0.09 mg/kg/day			NCBRF-hyperactive	Significant for	weight gain 13%, dyspepsia
8.1 ±2.3	6-week duration			NCBRF-overly sensitive	boys, not for girls	9%, increased appetite 5%
				NCBRF-isolated/	No change in	No SAE
				ritualistic	lab values except	
				NCBRF-self injury/	prolactin	
				stereotypic	No cognitive	
				ABC-irritability	changes	
				ABC-hyperactivity		
				ABC-social		
				withdrawal/lethargy		
				BPI-aggressive/		
				destructive		
				Nonsignificant results		
				ABC-stereotypy		
				ABC-inappropriate		
				Speech		
				CGI-C (equivalent to		
				CGI-I), % improved		
				BPI-self-injurious		
				BPI-stereotyped		

Continued

TABLE 3.2 Published Randomized Controlled Trials of SGAs for DBDs in Children and Adolescents—Cont'd

Lead Author, Year, Journal	n; % ♂; Age (Years): Range, Mean Age	Drug/Dose; Duration	Concurrent Medications	Primary Outcome#	Secondary Outcomes	Weight Change/ Metabolic Effects	Adverse Effects
Aman et al. (2014); J Am Acad Child Adolesc Psychiatry	n=168 77% ♂; Age range 6-12 R: 9.03±2.05 PBO: 8.75±1.98	Flexible dose§ (<25 kg, ≥25 kg) Mean 1.7±0.75 mg/ day 6-week duration	Methyl-phenidate R: 46.1±16.8 PBO: 44.8±14.6	NCBRF-D total R: 15.2** PBO: −7.1 ES 0.5 [Total D includes conduct problem and oppositional subscale]	*Statistically significant results* NCBRF-positive/ social ABS-reactive! *Nonsignificant results* ABS-proactive! NCBRF-ADHD NCBRF-overly sensitive NCBRF-withdrawn Responder: (>25% decrease on D score & CGI-I of 1 or 2) CGI-I (% improved) CGI-S %	*Weight change* R:+1.8±1 kg** PBO: − 1.2 ±2 kg *BMI percentile change* R: +0.4** PBO: −10.7 *Prolactin change* R: +30.1 μg/l** PBO: +1.4 μg/l *Abnormal lab results* R: n=2 (triglyceride 389mg/dL, prolactin 112 μg/L) PBO: n=2 (fasting glucose 144mg/ dL, fasting insulin 24 μIU/mL)	*Neurological* headache 1% *Gastrointestinal* decreased appetite 12%, stomach discomfort 11%, vomiting 6%, increased appetite 5%

Study	Sample	Dose	Prior medication	Efficacy results	Other results	Weight change	Adverse effects
Armenteros et al. (2007); J Am Acad Child Adolesc Psychiatry	n=25 88% ♂; Age range 7-12 R: 7.3±3.7 PBO: 8.8±3.1	Flexible dose Mean 1.08±0.63 mg/day 4-week duration	Required at least 3 weeks on stimulant medication prior to trial: methylphenidate (Range 18-54mg/day): 60%; mixed amphetamine salts (range 10-40mg/day): 40%	CAS-PARENT (% improved by 30%) R: 100%**; PBO: 77% No statistically significant difference on 4 individual subscales CAS-Teacher % improved by 30%: R: 27% PBO: 54% No statistically significant difference on 3 individual subscales	*Nonsignificant results* CGI-I CGI-S CPRS CTRS	*Weight change* R: +0.9±0.3 kg PBO: −0.06±0.4 kg No BMI changes, blood cell count, electrolytes, thyroid & kidney function, urinalyses remained normal in both groups	*Neurological* agitation 8% *Gastrointestinal* stomach pain 17%, increased appetite 8%
Buitelaar et al. (2001); J Clin Psychiatry	n=38 87% ♂; Age range 12-18 R: 14±1.5 PBO: 13.7±2	Flexible dose Mean 2.9±0.04 mg/kg/day Range 1.5-4 mg/day 6-week duration	*No information provided*	CGI-S R: −1.6**; PBO: 0.2 CGI-S % improved R: 58%***; PBO: −5%	*Statistically significant results* OAS-overall score (Wrd) OAS-aggression against property (Wrd) OAS physical aggression (Wrd) ABC-irritability (Sch/Wrd) ABC-hyperactivity (Sch/Wrd)	*Weight change* R: +2.3 kg** PBO: +0.6 kg No differences in hematologic or biochemical parameters (including liver function, electrolytes, thyroid function, blood pressure, heart rate, ECG, QTc)	*Any* 31% *Neurological* tiredness 53%, slowness 20%, headache 11%, somnolence 11%, fatigue 11%, tremor 9%, dizziness 5%, muscle stiffness 4%

Continued

TABLE 3.2 Published Randomized Controlled Trials of SGAs for DBDs in Children and Adolescents—Cont'd

Lead Author, Year, Journal	n; % δ; Age (Years): Range, Mean Age	Drug/Dose; Duration	Concurrent Medications	Primary Outcome#	Secondary Outcomes	Weight Change/ Metabolic Effects	Adverse Effects
					ABC-inappropriate speech (Sch/Wrd) ABC-stereotypy (Sch) *Nonsignificant results* OAS-verbal aggression (Sch/Wrd) OAS-auto aggression (Sch/Wrd) ABC-stereotypy (Wrd) ABC-social withdrawal/lethargy (Sch/Wrd) OAS-overall score (Sch) OAS-aggression against property (Sch) OAS-physical aggression (Sch)	*Prolactin change* R: +16.8 ng/ml** PBO: −5.4 ng/ml	*HEENT* sialorrhea 21%, difficulty swallowing/talking 21% *Gastrointestinal* nausea 16% SAE Notes: "R: 11% relapse of aggressive behavior PBO: 5% ran away and hospitalized for alcohol intoxication"

| Findling et al. (2000); J Am Acad Child Adolesc Psychiatry | n=20 95% δ; Age range 6-14 R: 10.7±3.4 PBO: 8.2±1.9 | Flexible dose§ <50 kg: 0.25 mg per tablet≥ 50 kg: 0.5 mg per tablet Mean: 4.1 tablets, 0.03 mg/kg/day Range 0.75-1.5 mg/day 10-week duration | No information provided | RAAPP R: −1.65** PBO: −0.16 | Statistically significant results CGI-S CGI-I CPRS conduct problems subscale CBCL delinquent behavior scale Nonsignificant results CPRS: Learning Problem, Psychosomatic, Impulsive-Hyperactive, Anxiety, and Hyperactivity scales CBCL: Withdrawn, Somatic Complaints, Anxious/Depressed, Social Problems, Thought Problems, Attention Problems and Aggressive Behavior subscales | Predicted weight change (accounting for dropouts) R: +4.2±0.7 kg** PBO: +0.8±0.9 kg No clinically significant changes in lab values or ECG, no parkinsonian symptoms or acute dystonic reaction | Any 40% Neurological sedation 10%, insomnia 10%, irritability 10%, restlessness 10% Gastrointestinal increased appetite 30% Dermatological rash 10% |

Continued

TABLE 3.2 Published Randomized Controlled Trials of SGAs for DBDs in Children and Adolescents—Cont'd

Lead Author, Year, Journal	n; % δ; Age (Years): Range, Mean Age	Drug/Dose; Duration	Concurrent Medications	Primary Outcome#	Secondary Outcomes	Weight Change/ Metabolic Effects	Adverse Effects
Snyder et al. (2002); J Am Acad Child Adolesc Psychiatry	n=110 76% δ; Age range 5–12 R: 8.6±0.26 PBO: 8.8±0.27	Flexible dose Mean 0.98±0.06 0.03 mg/kg/day Range: 0.4– 3.8 mg/day 6-week duration	No information provided	NCBRF-conduct problem R: −15.8** PBO: −6.8	*Statistically significant results* NCBRF-competent calm NCBRF-adaptive/social NCBRF-conduct problem NCBRF-insecure/ anxious NCBRF-hyperactive NCBRF-isolated/ ritualistic NCBRF-self injury/ stereotypic ABC-irritability ABC-hyperactivity ABC-stereotypy ABC-social withdrawal/lethargy ABC-inappropriate Speech BPI-aggressive/ destructive VAS-symptom CGI-1% *Nonsignificant results*	*Weight change* R: +2.2 kg** PBO: +0.2 kg *Prolactin change* R: +39 ng/ml** PBO: −2.25 ng/ml No clinically relevant mean changes hematologic, clinical chemistry, or urinalysis. QTc increases between 30 and 60 ms (R: 6% PBO 4%), increase 60+ (R 2%, PBO 2%). No ECGs clinically significant No difference in blood pressure Nonsignificant mean pulse rate change No changes on CPT or CVLT	*Any* 13% *Neurological* abnormal crying 8%, emotional lability 2%, headache 10%, somnolence 28%, fatigue 8%, hyperprolactinemia 11%, hypertonia 6% *HEENT* increased saliva 9% *Respiratory* cough 6%, epistaxis 9%, nasopharyngitis 4%, rhinitis 4% *Gastrointestinal* weight gain 8%, increased appetite 11%, anorexia 4%, vomiting 4%, dyspepsia 8% *Genitourinary* enuresis 8% *Dermatological* rash 6%

				Primary	Measures		
Van Bellinghen and deTroch (2001); *J Child Adolesc Psychopharmacol*	n=13 38% ♂; Age range 6-14 Median R:10.5 PBO:11	Flexible dose Mean 1.2 mg/day 0.05 mg/kg/day Range 0.03-0.06 mg/kg/day 4-week duration	Valproate 8%	*Primary Outcome not defined* ABC-Irritability R: −10.8** PBO: 0.1 ABC-Hyperactivity R: −14.8** PBO: 1 ABC-Stereotypy R: 0.7 PBO: −0.7 ABC-Social Withdrawal/Lethargy R: −1.7 PBO: −3.9** ABC-Inappropriate Speech R: −2.3 PBO: 0.1	NCBRF-overly sensitive BPI-self-injurious BPI-stereotyped *Significant Negative Effect* VAS-sedation *Primary Measures cont'd: Primary measure not defined; Statistically significant results* VAS-parent-rated most disturbing behavior PAC-social relationships PAC-occupational attitudes *Nonsignificant results* PAC-independence in personal care PAC-adaptation PAC-temperament PAC-sexual attitude PAC-communicativeness PAC-truthfulness	*Weight change* R: +1.8kg PBO: +0.6kg Statistically significant (but not clinically significant) increased heart rate for R (9.3 beats/min) after 3 weeks, no difference in blood pressure, no consistent changes in blood, hematology, or urinalysis	*Any* 15%

Continued

TABLE 3.2 Published Randomized Controlled Trials of SGAs for DBDs in Children and Adolescents—Cont'd

Lead Author, Year, Journal	n; % δ; Age (Years): Range, Mean Age	Drug/Dose; Duration	Concurrent Medications	Primary Outcome#	Secondary Outcomes	Weight Change/ Metabolic Effects	Adverse Effects
				CGI-I (end mean/% improved) R: −2.2** 83% PBO: −0.2, 0%	PAC-honesty PAC-responsiveness PAC-peer's attitudes PAC-cooperation PAC-dominance		

Abbreviations: A = aripiprazole; BMI = body mass index; EPS = extrapyramidal symptoms; ES = effect size; FBG = fasting blood glucose; HDL = high-density lipoprotein; HEENT = head, eyes, ears, nose, and throat; LDL = low-density lipoprotein; MPH = methylphenidate; N/A = not available; O = olanzapine; PBO = placebo; R = risperidone; SAE = serious adverse events; Sch: school rating; Tchol = total cholesterol; TG = triglyceride; URTI = upper respiratory tract infection; Wrd: ward rating; δ = male; † = positive score denotes improvement; ∧ = present in group, as other group details were missing; ** = statistically significant result; # primary outcome scores refer to "mean change from baseline."

Abbreviations of rating scales used: ABC-I: Aberrant Behavior Checklist (Irritability subscale); ABC: Aberrant Behavior Checklist; BPI: Behavior Problems Inventory; ABS: Antisocial Behavior Scale; CAS: Children's Aggression Scale; CARS: Childhood Autism Rating Scale; CBCL: Child Behavior Checklist; CDRS-R: Children's Depression Rating Scale-Revised; CGI-C: Clinical Global Impression-Change; CGI-I: Clinical Global Impression-Improvement; CGAS: Children's Global Assessment Scale; CMRS: Child Mania Rating Scale; CPRS: Conners Parent Rating Scale; CTRS: Conners Teacher Rating Scale; Caregiver Strain Questionnaire; cY-BOCS: Children's Yale-Brown Obsessive-Compulsive Scale; GARS: Gilliam Autism Rating Scale; KADS: Kutcher Adolescent Depression Scale; NCBRF: Nisonger Child Behavior Rating Form; OAS: Overt Aggression Scale; PAC: Personal Assessment Checklist; PedsQL: Pediatric Quality of Life Inventory; Q-LES-Q: Quality of Life Enjoyment & Satisfaction Questionnaire; RAAPP: Rating of Aggression Against People and/or Property Scale; SNAP-IV: Swanson, Nolan and Pelham Scale-Version IV; VABS: Vineland Adaptive Behavior Scale; VAS: Visual Analog Scale; YMRS: Young Mania Rating Scale.

Box 3.1   Summary of the Most Common Outcome Measures

ABC

The Aberrant Behavior Checklist (ABC; Aman, Singh, Stewart, & Field, 1985) is a 58-item parent/caregiver-rated scale of child behavior, which was designed to assess treatment effect rather than clinical outcome. It includes five subscales: Irritability, Social Withdrawal/Lethargy, Stereotypic Behavior, Hyperactivity, and Inappropriate Speech. Average scores by age and gender have been provided to anchor research scores (Aman et al., 1985).

CARS

The CARS (Schopler, Reichler, DeVellis, & Daly, 1980) is a 23-item, clinician-rated observation scale that is used in the diagnosis of ASD. It includes 14 domains assessing behaviors, and 1 domain of clinical impressions. Each domain is scored between 1 and 4, with an overall total score of 15-60. Scores of above 30 indicate autistic spectrum disorder, with a score of >37 indicating severe autism.

CGI

The Clinical Global Impressions Scale (CGI; Busner & Targum, 2007) is a clinician-rated scale that provides three scores, the CGI-Improvement/Change, CGI-Severity, and a therapeutic response item. Severity and Improvement are each assessed with one question on a seven-point scale (1 being normal/very much improved and 7 extremely ill/very much worse). Therapeutic response is assessed with a four-point scale.

cY-BOCS

The cY-BOCS (Scahill et al., 1997) is a diagnostic tool, which involves a semi-structured interview by a clinician with a parent. It contains an obsessions and compulsions checklist as well as a severity rating scale, and provides an overall total score which is rated as follows: 0-7 subclinical, 8-15 mild, 16-23 moderate, 24-31 severe, and 32-40 extreme OCD.

CMRS

The CMRS (Pavuluri, Henry, Devineni, Carbray, & Birmaher, 2006) is a 21-item screening tool completed by parents for the symptoms of mania. Responses are scored as follows: never = 0, sometimes = 1, often = 2, and very often = 3. A score of above 20 indicates that clinical advice should be sought.

NCBRF

The N-CBRF (Aman, Tassé, Rojahn, & Hammer, 1996) is a 76-item parent-completed measure of child behavior, specifically designed for children with developmental disabilities. Parents rate each behavior on a four-point scale. There are two Positive Social subscales (Compliant/Calm and Adaptive Social) and six Problem Behavior subscales (Conduct Problems, Insecure/Anxious, Hyperactive, Self-injury/Stereotypic, Self-Isolated/Ritualistic, and Overly sensitive). There is also a version to be completed by teachers. Age and gender normative scores are available (Norris & Lecavalier, 2011; Tasse, Aman, Hammer, & Rohan, 1996).

Box 3.2   Summary of Most Common Adverse Effects Measures

AIMS

The AIMS (Munetz & Benjamin, 1988) is a 12-item indirect observation scale of dyskinesia. The clinician rates patient orofacial movements, dental issues, and dyskinesia of body (limb and trunk), provides a clinical impression of severit y and asks for patient subjective judgment. The total score ranges from 0 to 42, however there is no consensus on cut off scores.

BARS

The BARS (Barnes, 1989) is an observation scale of the presence and frequency of drug-induced akathisia. Clinicians observe patients in seated and in standing positions and rate symptoms on a scale of 0 (normal) to −3 (constantly restless) and ask patients to give subjective ratings of restlessness and any related distress. Responses are combined to provide a Global Clinical Assessment of Akathisia, which ranges from 0 (akathisia absent/pseudoakathisia) to 5 (severe akathisia).

SAS

The Simpson Angus Scale (SAS; Hawley et al., 2003) is a performance scale that measures drug-induced parkinsonism symptoms. The rater asks the patient to perform 10 tasks and rates responses on a scale of 0-4 (normal to severe). Specific symptoms include muscle rigidity, tremor, reflexes, and salivation. A total score of 0-40 is calculated (or scale score can be calculated by dividing the total by 10 to give a score between 0 and 4), with a raw score of <3 identifying "normal" symptoms, ≥6 indicating a level of disorder for which treatment should be reconsidered, ≥12 requiring attention, and a score of ≥18 "almost certainly" requiring modification of pharmacotherapy (Hawley et al., 2003).

Three trials included only children less than 13 years of age, while the remainder included children 5-17 years of age. The mean age ranged from 4 to 10.2 years of age. Trial participants were overwhelmingly male (74-90% of the trial samples). Only half of the RCTs provided information on the level of intellectual disability (formerly called mental retardation) present in their sample. In those trials, between 52% and 81% of the trial sample were reported to have an intellectual disability. Further, four of the eight trials excluded children who were known to be treatment resistant to either the medication under study or antipsychotic drugs in general.

The majority of RCTs were of an 8-week duration, while two RCTs were 6 months long. There was one fixed-dose trial for aripiprazole with three dosage levels (5, 10, and 15 mg/day) and one flexible-dose trial, with a mean dosage of 8.9 mg/day (range: 2-15 mg/day). The lone olanzapine trial involved a flexible-dose design, with dosage based on body weight categories (above or below 40 kg). The mean overall olanzapine dose was 10 ± 2.04 mg/day, with a range of 7.5-12.5 mg/day. There were five risperidone RCTs, two with fixed-dose designs and three with flexible-dose designs. The 6-month trial by Nagaraj, Singhi, and

Malhi (2006) had a fixed dose of 1 mg/day, whereas Kent et al. (2013) included fixed high and low risperidone dosages, with body weight categories of above or below 45 kg. Thus, the fixed low dose was 0.125 and 0.175 mg/day, and the high dose was 1.25 and 1.75 mg/day, respectively. The three flexible-dose trials had final mean doses of 1.14 ± 0.32, 1.48, and 1.8 ± 0.7 mg/day respectively, within a range of 0.5-3.5 mg/day.

All eight RCTs were monotherapy trials. Participants received the study SGA or matching placebo only, without other drug treatments administered by the investigators. In Luby et al. (2006), applied behavioral analysis (ABA) therapy was concurrently employed for all patients as this treatment was mandated for all children in that geographical district. The treatment group received a mean of 21.2 h a week of ABA therapy while the placebo group received less, at a mean of 11.3 h per week. As an accepted intervention for children with ASD, this discrepancy may have confounded the treatment effects in the risperidone group. In Nagaraj et al. (2006), other psychoactive drugs were stopped at least a month prior to the start of the trial; 16% of the active treatment group and 5% of the placebo group had taken other antipsychotic medications, and conversely 5% of the active treatment group and 15% of the placebo group had been taking stimulant medication. Most studies provided detailed information on concurrent medications that the children were taking along with the study drug or placebo. For two of the three trials that did not provide this information, details were provided on which concurrent medications were allowed in the trial (for example, anticonvulsants, or clonidine or chloral hydrate for sleep).

Both aripiprazole studies used the Aberrant Behavior Checklist-Irritability subscale (ABC-I) as the primary outcome measure, with statistically significant treatment effects observed in both trials. Owen et al. (2009) reported a treatment effect size (Cohen's d) of 0.87, which is considered a large effect size. Similarly, statistically significant treatment effects were observed for the overall response rate, Clinical Global Impression-Improvement (CGI-I), Clinical Global Impression-Severity (CGI-S), Children's Yale-Brown Obsessive-Compulsive Scale (cY-BOCS) and the ABC Hyperactivity, Stereotypy and Inappropriate Speech subscales, although not for all dosage levels in the Marcus et al. (2009) trial. Statistically significant treatment effects were not observed on the ABC-Social Withdrawal scale in either trial, nor for the Pediatric Quality of Life Inventory (PedsQL) or Caregiver Strain Questionnaire (CGSQ) in the Owen et al. (2009) trial.

The CGI-I was the primary outcome measure in the olanzapine study, with a numerically higher, although non-statistically significant response rate in the treatment group (50%) compared with placebo (20%). Non-statistically significant treatment effects were observed on secondary measures of the cY-BOCS compulsion scale and the Overt Aggression Scale-Modified (OAS-M) irritability and aggression scales.

Three risperidone RCTs (Kent et al., 2013; RUPPAN, 2002; Shea et al., 2004) used the ABC-I as the primary outcome measure. Statistically significant treatment effects were reported in all three trials, although not for the low-dose risperidone group in the Kent et al. (2013) trial. The RUPPAN (2002) study reported a treatment effect size (Cohen's d) of 1.2, which is considered large to very large. The overall response rate in the RUPPAN trial was also statistically significant for risperidone over placebo. The Childhood Autism Rating Scale (CARS) was used as the primary outcome in the other two risperidone trials (Luby et al., 2006; Nagaraj et al., 2006). Statistically significant treatment effects were reported for both of these trials, as well as on the Children's Global Assessment Scale (CGAS) in Nagaraj et al. (2006). The Gilliam Autism Rating Scale (GARS), a primary outcome measure in the Luby et al. (2006) trial, was not found to be significantly different for risperidone compared to placebo in a time by treatment interaction.

Among secondary outcome measures, three trials reported results for the other ABC subscales. Statistically significant treatment effects results were observed on the ABC Hyperactivity and Stereotypy scales in all three trials, although not for the low-dose risperidone group in Kent et al. (2013) study. Mixed findings were observed on the ABC Social Withdrawal/Lethargy and Inappropriate Speech subscales. Positive treatment effects were observed on the CGI-I, CGI-S, cY-BOCS, Global Impressions Scale, and Nisonger Child Behavior Rating Form (N-CBRF) where measured, but not on the Child Behavior Checklist (CBCL) or Vineland Adaptive Behavior Scales (VABS).

Overall, SGAs were observed to have a positive treatment effect on the ABC-Irritability, Hyperactivity and Stereotypy scales as well as on overall clinical improvement for children with ASDs. Evidence for a positive treatment effect on the ABC Social Withdrawal/Lethargy scale and Compulsive behaviors was mixed.

Efficacy of SGAs for Children and Adolescents With DBDs

Nine RCTs which compared SGAs to placebo for treatment of DBD symptoms were identified, one with aripiprazole, one with quetiapine, and seven with risperidone. No RCTs for treatment of DBDs were identified for asenapine, clozapine, lurasidone, olanzapine, paliperidone, or ziprasidone. A summary of these RCTs can be found in Table 3.2. In contrast to the ASD trials where all but two trials provided details of when the trial was conducted, only two of the DBD trials provided this information (between 2003 and 2007). All trials were published between 2000 and 2014; five trials were conducted in the United States, one in Brazil, one in Netherlands, one in Belgium, and one in multiple countries (United States, Canada, and South Africa). The number of treatment sites per trial ranged between 1 and 16 sites. In eight of the nine trials, funding for the study was provided, at least in part, by the pharmaceutical company that manufactured the SGA studied.

A range of diagnostic categories were included in these trials, including CD, ODD ADHD, and ADHD co-morbid with pediatric bipolar disorder, with a variety of measures used to determine symptom severity for inclusion (for example, a CGI-S score ≥ 4 or an N-CBRF≥ 24). Some trials specified that a sub-average intelligence quotient (IQ) was a requirement for inclusion (Aman et al., 2002; Buitelaar, van der Gaag, Cohen-Kettenis, & Melman, 2001; Snyder et al., 2002; Van Bellinghen & deTroch, 2001) while others excluded youth with an IQ below 75 (and/or mild intellectual disability) and subsequently reported the average IQ of the groups (Aman et al., 2014; Armenteros, Lewis, & Davalos, 2007; Tramontina et al., 2009). A single trial reported that treatment resistance to risperidone was part of the exclusion criteria (Armenteros et al., 2007). In contrast to the ASD trials, most of DBD trials involved a lead-in period of 1-3 weeks to account for placebo responders (Connor, McLaughlin, & Jeffers-Terry 2008; Snyder et al., 2002) and standard treatment responders (Aman et al., 2014; Armenteros et al., 2007; Buitelaar et al., 2001) prior to randomization. Standard ADHD treatment was concurrent with risperidone in both the Aman et al. (2014) and Armenteros et al. (2007) trials, specifically methylphenidate (mean 45.45 mg/day, range 18-54 mg/day) or mixed amphetamine salts (range 10-40 mg/day). Parent training was also concurrent in the Aman et al. (2014) trial.

The RCTs ranged in size, from 13 to 168 participants (total 554) and most applied an ITT analysis. Four trials included only children less than 13 years of age (Aman et al., 2002, 2014; Armenteros et al., 2007; Snyder et al., 2002), two trials included only adolescents 12-18 years of age (Buitelaar et al., 2001; Connor et al., 2008), while the remaining three trials included youth from 6 to 17 years of age. The mean ages ranged from 7.3 to 15 years of age. The proportion of males was higher (74-95%) in most trials, except for Tramontina et al. (2009; 47% male) and Van Bellinghen and deTroch (2001; 38% male).

Trials were 4-10 weeks duration, and most involved a flexible-dose design. The aripiprazole trial had a body weight consideration for dosing (above or below 50 kg), with a mean dose of 13.61 ± 5.37 mg/day (range 5-20 mg/day). The quetiapine trial was also flexible dose, with a mean of 294 ± 78 mg/day (range 200-600 mg/day). The seven risperidone trials had a flexible-dose design with mean dosages ranging between 0.63 and 2.9 mg/day. Aman et al. (2014) and Findling et al. (2000) included dose categories based on body weight; above or below 25 kg and above or below 50 kg, respectively. Five trials reported the mean risperidone dose per kg per day, with a range of 0.03-0.05 mg/kg/day.

The CGI-I, CGI-S, and NCBRF were the most common outcome measures used in the DBD trials, although there was a great deal of variety in the measures used, with trials administering between four and five outcome measures, some with up to eight subscales each. The aripiprazole study reported a positive treatment effect on the Young Mania Rating Scale (YMRS) but not on the SNAP-IV (which measures ADHD symptoms). Among the secondary outcomes, there was a positive treatment effect for the Child Mania Rating Scale (CRMS) and

CGI-S but not for either of the depression scales. The quetiapine trial reported positive treatment effects on the CGI-I and CGI-S, and on the Quality of Life Enjoyment & Satisfaction Questionnaire (Q-LES-Q) secondary measure, but not on the Overt Aggression Scale (OAS) total score or the Conners Parent Rating Scale (CPRS).

There was little consistency across the measures reported in the risperidone trials. All primary outcomes, however, demonstrated some positive treatment effects, including NCBRF-conduct problem, NCBRF-D total, CAS-parent scale, CGI-S, CGI-I, RAAPP, VAS, and most ABC subscales. The primary outcomes that were not found to be positively significant were the CAS-Teacher scale (Armenteros et al., 2007) and the ABC-Inappropriate Speech subscale (Van Bellinghen & deTroch, 2001). Further, there was a negative treatment effect for the ABC-Social Withdrawal/Lethargy subscale in the Van Bellinghen and deTroch (2001) trial.

There were mixed results among the secondary outcome measures, with positive treatment effects on the CGI-I and CGI-S observed in some trials (Findling et al., 2000; Snyder et al., 2002) but not others (Armenteros et al., 2007). Similarly, there were positive treatment effects on the ABC-Stereotypy and Inappropriate Speech subscales in one trial (Snyder et al., 2002) but not in others (Buitelaar et al., 2001; Van Bellinghen & deTroch, 2001). All other ABC subscales were reported to have statistically significant treatment effects. Both Aman et al. (2002) and Snyder et al. (2002) reported positive treatment effects on the aggression subscale of the Behavior Problems Inventory (BPI), but not on the self-injury or stereotypy scales. There was a statistically significant increase in the Visual Analog Scale (VAS) sedation scale, indicating increased levels of sedation in the risperidone treatment group.

Summary of Adverse Effects and Safety Data from ASD and DBD Trials Combined

Wide variance in the reporting of adverse effects was observed, with some studies reporting all adverse effects and others only reporting those present in at least 5% or 10% of a group. Thus, for potential adverse effects when no data was provided it is unclear whether these were not present or not measured. Overall, however, the abnormal involuntary movement scale (AIMS), Barnes Akathisia rating scale (BARS), and the Simpson-Angus Scale (SAS), used to evaluate extrapyramidal symptoms (EPS), were widely cited as tools to collect adverse effect data. The adverse effects columns in Tables 3.1 and 3.2 contain information about the reported adverse effects that were present in the SGA treatment groups, and percentages signify the percentage of participants in the SGA group reporting this effect, minus the percentage of participants in the placebo group reporting the same effect.

In the three aripiprazole RCTs (across both ASD and DBD trials), EPS, tremor, and fatigue/tiredness were among the most commonly reported adverse effects. Akathisia (restlessness) is an adverse effect of aripiprazole that is commonly reported in schizophrenia and bipolar disorder RCTs with aripiprazole; however, this was not a frequently reported adverse effect in the aripiprazole ASD and DBD trials. Drooling and weight gain were reported with quetiapine, while sedation, constipation, and weight gain were reported adverse effects of olanzapine. There were 12 trials involving risperidone, and there was a wide variation in the adverse effects reported. Reports of "any" adverse effects ranged from −20% (i.e., 20% more participants in the placebo group reported adverse effects than the risperidone group) to 40%. Tremor, EPS, headache, sedation, somnolence, upper respiratory tract infections (URTIs), and hypersalivation/drooling were among the most commonly reported adverse effects across all four SGAs studied.

Overall, by body system, neurological adverse effects were the most commonly reported, including affect and movement problems. Gastrointestinal and respiratory effects were also common, including appetite changes and rhinitis. There were few cardiac adverse effects, however genitourinary effects (specifically enuresis) and dermatological issues were frequent.

The U.S. FDA describes serious adverse effects (SAEs) as any side effect caused by a medical product that is life threatening pr results in hospitalization or permanent damage (U.S. FDA, 2014). In the trials, SAEs were reported infrequently, with suicide-related behavior reported for the placebo (three reports) and aripiprazole (one report) groups in Owen et al. (2009), oligomenorrhea in the high-dose risperidone group in Kent et al. (2013), relapse of aggressive behavior in Buitelaar et al. (2001), and severe hyperkinesia/somnolence, aggressive reaction, and EPS for the risperidone group in Shea et al. (2004). Full details regarding SAEs are presented in Tables 3.1 and 3.2.

The majority of trials measured body weight and body mass index (BMI), while some reported prolactin changes along with other metabolic effects. None of the RCTs employed methods to account for normal weight gain through growth, and none used BMI z-scores (standard deviations from the mean) to determine if BMI change outpaced that expected with normal growth. Body weight was significantly increased compared to placebo for all three aripiprazole trials, yet BMI was not. While prolactin level elevation is commonly observed in practice with older first-generation antipsychotics and risperidone, both Marcus et al. (2009) and Owen et al. (2009) reported statistically significant reductions in prolactin levels in the aripiprazole treatment groups, while prolactin levels were not measured in Tramontina et al. (2009). There were no significant differences in other lab tests, including lipoprotein levels, fasting blood glucose, and cholesterol levels. Hollander et al. (2006) reported statistically significant weight gain for the olanzapine group compared to placebo, while quetiapine was not associated with a statistically significant difference for weight change or BMI or prolactin levels when compared to placebo. A higher than average pulse rate was reported in the quetiapine treatment group (Connor et al., 2008).

In 8 of the 12 risperidone trials, a statistically significant difference in weight was reported for the risperidone treatment groups compared to placebo, and while only 4 trials reported BMI, only Aman et al. (2014) reported a statistically significant difference for risperidone compared to placebo. Four of the six trials that reported prolactin levels indicated a significant increase for risperidone over placebo, and Aman et al. (2002) found a significant difference for boys, but not girls. The majority of other measurements did not result in statistically significant differences between treatment arms. Aman et al. (2014) reported abnormal results for triglycerides and prolactin for both the risperidone and placebo groups, while Van Bellinghen and deTroch (2001), Shea et al. (2004), and Snyder et al. (2002) all reported cardiac effects (increased heart rate and QTc interval).

DISCUSSION

SGAs Included in RCTs

Risperidone is the most studied SGA in children for treatment of ASDs and DBDs, with 12 of 17 RCTs identified during this review pertaining to risperidone. In other therapeutic domains such as schizophrenia and bipolar disorder, risperidone is also commonly used. A large part of the reason for the disproportional number of studies involving risperidone is that it was the first SGA to market, other than clozapine. Due to the risk for agranulocytosis (a severe deficiency of infection-fighting granulocytes, or neutrophils, in the blood) clozapine use has been restricted and extra monitoring is required. In North America, this rare but potentially fatal adverse effect sharply limits clozapine prescribing to only approved indications of schizophrenia and schizoaffective disorder, and only after two other antipsychotic trials are undertaken. These risks and precautions along with its high adverse effect burden make clozapine an unsuitable candidate for treatment of ASDs and DBDs. Risperidone was still under U.S. patent protection when the BPCA, with its incentivization of pediatric medication trials, was signed into law in 2002. Risperidone was the first SGA to obtain FDA approval for treatment of irritability of autism in 2006, followed by aripiprazole in 2009.

No RCTs for ASDs or DBDs were identified involving asenapine, clozapine, lurasidone, paliperidone, or ziprasidone. Other than clozapine (see reasons limiting its use detailed above), the other four drugs are relative newcomers to the SGA market, with market release dates subsequent to publication of the bulk of the RCT data detailed in this chapter. Despite the lack of regulatory approval in Canada, risperidone and aripiprazole are in some ways now considered established treatments for ASDs and DBDs, and there may be less clinical interest in studying the newer SGAs for these indications. Risperidone is now available in generic formulations in both Canada and the United States, and the drug cost is a fraction of that of branded treatments still under patent protection such as aripiprazole and other newer SGAs.

Efficacy in ASD Trials

A majority of SGA trials for treatment of ASDs examine response on the ABC irritability subscale (ABC-I) as the primary outcome measure, with most studies reporting positive treatment effects, often with large effect sizes (effect size is a method of expressing how noticeable the differences are between treatment groups). Treatment response on core symptoms of ASD (communication difficulties, social challenges, and repetitive behaviors) as measured by other ABC subscales was more variable. Trials using the CARS and GARS rating scales as primary outcome measures (Luby et al., 2006; Nagaraj et al., 2006) are difficult to compare to the trials using the ABC-I scale, since the CARS and GARS appear to measure more of the core autism symptoms, as opposed to irritability symptoms alone.

Only the olanzapine pilot trial failed to show a statistically significant treatment effect, although the number of subjects was very low ($n = 11$), making the trial underpowered statistically to show a difference between groups, with the possibility of a type II statistical error being made (i.e., failing to observe a difference between groups when one actually exists). No published head-to-head study comparing aripiprazole and risperidone for treatment of ASDs exists. However, this type of trial design is rarely seen in any pharmacotherapeutic area. While this information is strongly desired by clinicians to help with prescribing decisions, there is little to gain and potentially much to lose for pharmaceutical companies (particularly if their drug is found to be inferior) to participate in head-to-head comparison trials. To gain regulatory approval, companies only need to demonstrate superiority over placebo. Clinical trials are very expensive to conduct, and in a recent review it was found that 85-90% of clinical trials are funded by the drug's manufacturer (LaMattina, 2013). When head-to-head comparison studies do exist, they are typically funded by large public institutions such as the National Institute of Health, often several years after a drug is initially marketed. Without such data, comparing data from separate clinical trials is, at best, an apples-to-oranges comparison.

Of the ASDs trials, the RUPPAN (2002) risperidone trial and the Owen et al. (2009) aripiprazole trial were the most comparable in terms of design: approximately 100 subjects, more than 80% males, mean age of approximately 9 years of age, flexible dose, 8-week duration, and use of ABC-I as the primary outcome measure. The reported effect size was numerically larger in the risperidone trial (1.2, considered large to very large) than the reported effect size in the aripiprazole trial (0.87, considered large). However, there was a potentially significant difference at baseline, as patients had higher baseline symptom scores in the aripiprazole trial (mean 29.9) than the risperidone trial (mean 25.9). It is possible that treatment with aripiprazole in a population with more severe symptoms at baseline caused the effect size to appear smaller and underestimated what it might have been in a less severely ill cohort of patients, like those enrolled in the risperidone trial.

It should be mentioned that SGAs are not the sole available effective treatment for irritability of ASDs. Behavioral and nonpharmacological treatments are often employed, and should be continued even if treatment with an SGA or other pharmacotherapy is started (Frazier, 2012). Alternate medications with published RCT evidence to support efficacy in treatment of irritability of ASDs include anticonvulsants (valproate and topiramate), stimulants such as methylphenidate, the antihistamine cyproheptadine, and perhaps less obvious choices such as memantine, galantamine, and pentoxifylline (Elbe & Lalani, 2012; Ghaleiha et al., 2013).

Efficacy in DBD trials

Published evidence to date from RCTs points to an apparent benefit from SGA use for DBDs in children and youth. A closer examination warrants a cautious interpretation of the evidence supporting the use of SGAs in this population. This includes a very limited number of RCTs, essentially all focused on studying risperidone (seven out of nine trials), with inclusion of a wide range of symptoms, subject ages, and variations in cognitive capacities and use of outcome measures, as well as diagnostic confusion stemming from inclusion of trials studying pediatric bipolar disorder. Moreover, study designs that excluded SGA-treatment-resistant subjects or placebo responders prior to randomization may have "stacked the deck" in the direction of an outcome favoring SGA treatment. The inclusion of standard ADHD treatment (methylphenidate), wide ranges of RCT participant numbers across studies, variable treatment durations, and variations in outcome measures detracts from systematic comparisons across studies. Overall functioning and conduct/aggressive behaviors were found to be positively impacted by SGA treatment; however, stereotypies, social withdrawal, and depressive symptoms were less consistently improved. The wide range of measures and definitions of disruptive behavior along with the variety in sample sizes preclude a more definitive understanding of the potential treatment effects; however, there are indications that SGAs can alleviate disruptive behavior symptoms for children experiencing clinically significant difficulties.

While there is evidence supporting the efficacy of SGAs over placebo for the treatment of behavioral disorders associated with ASDs and DBDs, these benefits do not come without drawbacks. All trials reviewed showed significant weight gains associated with SGA use and most reported clinically significant metabolic adverse effects (increased triglycerides and prolactin levels). While there is some evidence that people with ASDs are at higher risk for metabolic adverse effects (De Hert, Dobbelaere, Sheridan, Cohen, & Correll, 2011) due to the small number of trials with children, the adverse effects data have been summarized here across both the ASDs and DBDs trials.

Critique and Ethical Considerations

This review of the available evidence must be considered within the context of RCTs involving pediatric populations, publication pathways, and funding sources. With 16 of 17 RCTs identified in this review reporting statistically significant treatment effects on primary outcome measures and 14 trials reporting manufacturer funding, it is recognized that there may be some publication bias against trials with negative findings. Seven of the 17 trials were published prior to the International Committee of Medical Journal Editors (ICMJE) 2005 decision that no clinical trials will be considered for publication unless they are included in a public clinical trials registry prior to commencing patient enrollment. Prior to this time, it was possible for pharmaceutical manufacturers to suppress publication of negative clinical trial data, since the data were held in-house and there was no publicly available source to confirm the existence of any given clinical trial. For example, GlaxoSmithKline conducted three clinical trials that evaluated the serotonin reuptake inhibitor paroxetine for treatment of depression in adolescents. When results from the three trials were pooled, paroxetine was found to be no more effective than placebo, and the company attempted to suppress release of this data to prevent a decline in sales. Eventually, this matter was settled as part of a larger combined criminal and civil case in 2012, and GlaxoSmithKline agreed to pay a $3 billion fine (Marshall, 2004; Waters, 2012).

Since some of the RCTs identified in our review were conducted in the early 2000s before the mandatory registry enrollment requirement, it is possible that some early trials in these therapeutic areas with negative findings were not published, and that the 17 RCTs identified in this chapter do not comprise the entire data set for the use of SGAs to treat of ASDs and DBDs. It is beyond the scope of this chapter to compare the published studies with those registered.

While there is some open-label extension data for SGAs in these therapeutic areas, there remains a lack of long-term trials overall to provide long-term safety and efficacy data. In clinical practice, once an SGA is started for treatment of these conditions, the duration of use often extends well beyond the typical 8-week duration evaluated in clinical trials, more often extending to month or years. This dissonance between trial length and prescribing practices should be recognized by prescribers and shared with family members. The short duration of these trials may also cause clinicians to underestimate the adverse effect burden of using SGAs for treatment of these conditions over longer durations.

The 17 trials portray a plethora of adverse effects; however, there are few clear patterns. Moreover, metabolic adverse effects were not well characterized in many RCTs, especially for trials published in the early 2000s, prior to development of clinical awareness regarding the high potential for serious metabolic adverse effects with SGAs in children and adolescents. Without an increase in RCT-based evidence confirming benefits for children with ASDs and DBDs, close monitoring of all children and adolescents taking SGAs for metabolic adverse effects is recommended, in accordance with current published Canadian guidelines (Pringsheim, Panagiotopoulos, Davidson, Ho, & Canadian Alliance for Monitoring Effectiveness and Safety of Antipsychotics in Children (CAMESA) guideline group, 2011).

There is perceived tension between pharmaceutical industry objectives (to sell products for profit) and public health needs, and mistrust is frequent. This is compounded by the role pharmaceutical companies play in drug development and trials, as their financial resources allows them to develop new and better drugs. A family living with a child who has complex behavioral needs may become overwhelmed by extreme views regarding antipsychotic medication, either anti-treatment due to a fear of adverse effects, or pro-treatment with unrealistic expectations of benefit. It is the role of healthcare professionals to bridge this complex discussion, providing families with information about what is known about the effectiveness and safety of off-label treatments, based on available evidence and tempered by clinical experience. The goal of this chapter is to provide a transparent, easy-to-read summary of the available evidence and allow the reader to think critically about this issue.

CONCLUSION

While SGAs for use in children with ASD and DBDs lack formal regulatory approval from Health Canada, the majority of the available published RCT evidence supports the efficacy of certain SGAs (aripiprazole and risperidone for irritability associated with ASDs, and aripiprazole, risperidone, and quetiapine for DBDs). However, there are limitations to the evidence base. More than two-thirds of published RCTs identified were for risperidone, likely by virtue of it being the first (non-clozapine) SGA to market, rather than from any expectation of superior efficacy. Significant heterogeneity in outcome measures was observed, especially in DBD trials, and methodological variations distract from solid evidence of the efficacy of SGAs in this context. More RCTs of longer duration with consistent outcome and adverse effect evaluation parameters are desired to solidify the evidence base and to provide more relevant information about potential safety issues, so that clinicians can fully inform patients and families of the potential risks and benefits of these medications. Evaluation of newer SGAs (some of which have shown a reduced metabolic adverse effect profile in adults in RCTs) for these therapeutic areas would be welcomed.

REFERENCES

Alessi-Severini, S., Biscontri, R. G., Collins, D. M., Sareen, J., & Enns, M. A. (2012). Ten years of antipsychotic prescribing to children: A Canadian population based study. *Canadian Journal of Psychiatry, 57*, 52–58.

Aman, M. G., Singh, N. N., Stewart, A. W., & Field, C. J. (1985). The Aberrant Behavior Checklist: A behavior rating scale for the assessment of treatment effects. *American Journal of Mental Deficiency, 89*, 485–491.

Aman, M. G., Tassé, M. J., Rojahn, J., & Hammer, D. (1996). The Nisonger CBRF: A Child Behavior Rating Form for children with developmental disabilities. *Research in Developmental Disabilities, 17*, 41–57.

American Psychiatric Association. (2013). *Diagnostic and statistical manual of mental disorders* (5th ed.). Arlington, VA: American Psychiatric Publishers.

Barnes, T. R. (1989). A rating scale for drug-induced akathisia. *British Journal of Psychiatry, 154*, 672–676.

Belluz, J. (2012). *Psychotropes and children: Are we ruining a generation?* http://www.macleans.ca/authors/julia-belluz/psychotropes-and-children-ruining-a-generation/, Accessed March 30, 2014.

Busner, J., & Targum, S. D. (2007). The clinical global impressions scale: Applying a research tool in clinical practice. *Psychiatry, 4*, 28–37.

Chance, M. (2013). *Chemical lobotomies: A growing number of children are being prescribed antipsychotics for ADHD.* http://www.naturalnews.com/039742_chemical_lobotomy_antipsychotics_adhd.html, Accessed March 30, 2014.

De Hert, M., Dobbelaere, M., Sheridan, E. M., Cohen, D., & Correll, C. U. (2011). Metabolic and endocrine adverse effects of second-generation antipsychotics in children and adolescents: A systematic review of randomized, placebo controlled trials and guidelines for clinical practice. *European Psychiatry, 26*, 144–158.

Elbe, D., & Lalani, Z. (2012). Review of the pharmacotherapy of irritability of autism. *Journal of the Canadian Academy of Child and Adolescent Psychiatry, 21*, 130–146.

Frazier, T. W. (2012). Friends not foes: Combined risperidone and behavior therapy for irritability in autism. *Journal of the American Academy of Child and Adolescent Psychiatry, 51*, 129–131.

Ghaleiha, A., Ghyasvand, M., Mohammadi, M. R., Farokhnia, M., Yadegari, N., Tabrizi, M., et al. (2013). Galantamine efficacy and tolerability as an augmentative therapy in autistic children: A randomized, double-blind, placebo-controlled trial. *Journal of Psychopharmacology, 28*, 677–685.

Harrison, J. N., Cluxton-Keller, F., & Gross, D. (2012). Antipsychotic medication prescribing trends in children and adolescents. *Journal of Pediatric Health Care, 26*, 139–145.

Hawley, C. J., Finberg, N., Roberts, A. G., Baldwin, D., Sahadevan, A., & Sharman, V. (2003). The use of the Simpson Angus Scale for the assessment of movement disorder: A training guide. *International Journal of Psychiatry in Clinical Practice, 7*, 249–257.

Jacobson, R. (2014). *Should children take antipsychotic drugs?* http://www.scientificamerican.com/article/should-children-take-antipsychotic-drugs/, Accessed March 30, 2014.

Janssen Pharmaceuticals Inc. Risperdal (risperidone). (2013). Highlights of prescribing information. Titusville, NJ. http://www.janssenpharmaceuticalsinc.com/assets/risperdal.pdf, Accessed March 30, 2014

King, C., & Voruganti, L. N. (2002). What's in a name? The evolution of the nomenclature of antipsychotic drugs. *Journal of Psychiatry and Neuroscience, 27*, 168–175.

Kirkey, S. (2013). *Dramatic growth in antipsychotic drug even targets infants, experts say.* http://www.canada.com/health/Dramatic%2Bgrowth%2Bantipsychotic%2Bdrug%2Beven%2Btargets%2Binfants%2Bexperts/8407086/story.html, Accessed March 30, 2014.

LaMattina, J. (2013). Pharma controls clinical trials of their drugs. Is this hazardous to your health? *Forbes*, http://www.forbes.com/sites/johnlamattina/2013/10/02/pharma-controls-clinical-trials-of-their-drugs-is-this-hazardous-to-your-health/, Accessed September 5, 2014.

Marshall, E. (2004). Antidepressants and children. Buried data can be hazardous to a company's health. *Science, 304*, 1576–1577.

Moreno, C., Laje, G., Blanco, C., Jiang, H., Schmidt, A. B., & Olfson, M. (2007). National trends in the outpatient diagnosis and treatment of bipolar disorder in youth. *Archives of General Psychiatry, 64*, 1032–1039.

Munetz, M. R., & Benjamin, S. (1988). How to examine patients using the Abnormal Involuntary Movements Scale. *Hospital and Community Psychiatry, 39*, 1172–1177.

Norris, M., & Lecavalier, L. (2011). Evaluating the validity of the Nisonger Child Behavior Rating Form—Parent version. *Research in Developmental Disabilities, 32*, 2894–2900.

Olfson, M., He, J. P., & Merikangas, K. R. (2013). Psychotropic medication treatment of adolescents: Results from the national comorbidity survey-adolescent supplement. *Journal of the American Academy Child and Adolescent Psychiatry, 52*, 378–388.

Otsuka Pharmaceutical Co. Abilify (aripiprazole). (2013). *Highlights of prescribing information.* Tokyo, Japan: Otsuka Pharmaceutical. http://www.otsuka-us.com/Documents/Abilify.PI.pdf, Accessed March 30, 2014.

Pavuluri, M. N., Henry, D. B., Devineni, B., Carbray, J. A., & Birmaher, B. (2006). Child mania rating scale: Development, reliability and validity. *Journal of the American Academy of Child and Adolescent Psychiatry, 45*, 550–560.

Pringsheim, T., Panagiotopoulos, C., Davidson, J., Ho, J., & Canadian Alliance for Monitoring Effectiveness and Safety of Antipsychotics in Children (CAMESA) guideline group. (2011). Evidence-based recommendations for monitoring safety of second-generation antipsychotics in children and youth. *Journal of the Canadian Academy of Child and Adolescent Psychiatry, 20*(3), 218–233.

Reinberg, S. (2012). *More kids taking antipsychotics for ADHD: Study.* http://consumer.healthday.com/mental-health-information-25/behavior-health-news-56/more-kids-taking-antipsychotics-for-adhd-study-667425.html, Accessed March 30, 2014.

Ronsley, R., Scott, D., Warburton, W. P., Hamdi, R. D., Louie, D. C., Davidson, J., et al. (2013). A population-based study of antipsychotic prescription trends in children and adolescents in British Columbia, from 1996 to 2011. *Canadian Journal of Psychiatry, 58*, 361–369.

Scahill, L., Riddle, M. A., McSwiggin-Hardin, M., Ort, S. I., King, R. A., Goodman, W. K., et al. (1997). Children's Yale-Brown Obsessive-Compulsive Scale: Reliability and validity. *Journal of the American Academy of Child and Adolescent Psychiatry, 36*, 844–852.

Schopler, E., Reichler, R. J., DeVellis, R. F., & Daly, K. (1980). Toward objective classification of childhood autism: Childhood Autism Rating Scale (CARS). *Journal of Autism and Developmental Disorders, 10*, 91–103.

Swann, A. C. (2003). Neuroreceptor mechanisms of aggression and its treatment. *Journal of Clinical Psychiatry, 64*(Suppl. 4), 26–35.

Tasse, M. J., Aman, M. G., Hammer, D., & Rohan, J. (1996). The Nisonger Child Behavior Rating Form: Age and gender effects and norms. *Developmental Disabilities, 17*, 59–75.

Therapeutics Initiative. (2009). Increasing use of newer antipsychotics in children: A cause for concern? April-June 2009 *Therapeutics Newsletter, 74*, 1–2. http://www.ti.ubc.ca/sites/ti.ubc.ca/files/74.pdf, Accessed March 30, 2014.

U.S. Food and Drug Administration. (2002). *Best pharmaceuticals for children act.* Washington, DC: U.S. Food and Drug Administration. http://www.fda.gov/RegulatoryInformation/Legislation/FederalFoodDrugandCosmeticActFDCAct/SignificantAmendmentstotheFDCAct/ucm148011.htm, Accessed March 30, 2014.

U.S. Food and Drug Administration. (2014). *What is a serious adverse event?* http://www.fda.gov/safety/medwatch/howtoreport/ucm053087.htm, Accessed September 11, 2014.

Tusaie, K. R. (2010). Is the tail wagging the dog in pediatric bipolar disorder? *Archives of Psychiatric Nursing, 24*, 438–439.

Vitiello, B., Correll, C., van Zwieten-Boot, B., Zuddas, A., Parellada, M., & Arango, C. (2009). Antipsychotics in children and adolescents: Increasing use, evidence for efficacy and safety concerns. *European Neuropsychopharmacology, 19*, 629–635.

Waters, R. (2012). GlaxoSmithKline's $3 Billion Hit: Deterrent or Business Expense? *Forbes*, http://www.forbes.com/sites/robwaters/2012/07/12/glaxosmithklines-3-billion-hit-deterrent-or-business-expense/, Accessed September 5, 2014.

ASD STUDIES: ARIPIPRAZOLE

Marcus, R. N., Owen, R., Kamen, L., Manos, G., McQuade, R. D., Carson, W. H., et al. (2009). A placebo-controlled, fixed-dose study of aripiprazole in children and adolescents with irritability associated with autistic disorder. *Journal of the American Academy of Child and Adolescent Psychiatry, 48*, 1110–1119.

Owen, R., Sikich, L., Marcus, R. N., Corey-Lisle, P., Manos, G., McQuade, R. D., et al. (2009). Aripiprazole in the treatment of irritability in children and adolescents with autistic disorder. *Pediatrics, 124*, 1533–1540.

ASD STUDIES: OLANZAPINE

Hollander, E., Wasserman, S., Swanson, E. N., Chaplin, W., Schapiro, M. L., Zagursky, K., et al. (2006). A double-blind placebo-controlled pilot study of olanzapine in childhood/adolescent pervasive developmental disorder. *Journal of Child and Adolescent Psychopharmacology, 16*, 541–548.

ASD STUDIES: RISPERIDONE

Kent, J. M., Kushner, S., Xiaoping, N., Karcher, K., Ness, S., Aman, M., et al. (2013). Risperidone dosing in children and adolescents with autistic disorder: A double-blind placebo-controlled study. *Journal of Autism and Developmental Disorders, 43*, 1773–1783.

Luby, J., Mrakotsky, C., Stalets, M. M., Belden, A., Heffelfinger, A., Williams, M., et al. (2006). Risperidone in preschool children with autistic spectrum disorders: An investigation of safety and efficacy. *Journal of Child and Adolescent Psychopharmacology, 16*, 575–587.

Nagaraj, R., Singhi, P., & Malhi, P. (2006). Risperidone in children with autism: Randomized, placebo-controlled, double-blind study. *Journal of Child Neurology, 21*, 450–455.

Research Units on Pediatric Psychopharmacology Autism Network (RUPPAN). (2002). Risperidone in children with autism and serious behavioral problems. *The New England Journal of Medicine, 347*, 314–321.

Shea, S., Turgay, A., Carroll, A., Schulz, M., Orlik, H., Smith, I., et al. (2004). Risperidone in the treatment of disruptive behavioral symptoms in children with autistic and other pervasive developmental disorders. *Pediatrics, 114*, e634–e641.

DBD STUDIES: ARIPIPRAZOLE

Tramontina, S., Zeni, C. P., Ketzer, C. R., Pheula, G. F., Narvaez, J., & Rohde, L. A. (2009). Aripiprazole in children and adolescents with bipolar disorder comorbid with attention-deficit/hyperactivity disorder: A pilot randomized clinical trial. *Journal of Clinical Psychiatry, 70*, 756–764.

DBD STUDIES: QUETIAPINE

Connor, D. F., McLaughlin, T. J., & Jeffers-Terry, M. (2008). Randomized controlled pilot study of quetiapine in the treatment of adolescent conduct disorder. *Journal of Child and Adolescent Psychopharmacology, 18*, 140–156.

DBD STUDIES: RISPERIDONE

Aman, M. G., Bukstein, O. G., Gadow, K. D., Arnold, L. E., Molina, B. S. G., McNamara, N. K., et al. (2014). What does risperidone add to parent training and stimulant for severe aggression in child attention-deficit/hyperactivity disorder? *Journal of the American Academy of Child and Adolescent Psychiatry, 53*, 47–61.

Aman, M. G., de Smedt, G., Derivan, A., Lyons, B., Findling, R. L., Risperidone disruptive behavior study group. (2002). Double-blind, placebo-controlled study of risperidone for the treatment of disruptive behaviors in children with subaverage intelligence. *American Journal of Psychiatry, 159*, 1337–1346.

Armenteros, J. L., Lewis, J. E., & Davalos, M. (2007). Risperidone augmentation for treatment-resistant aggression in attention-deficit/hyperactivity disorder: A placebo-controlled pilot study. *Journal of the American Academy of Child and Adolescent Psychiatry, 46*, 558–565.

Buitelaar, J. K., van der Gaag, R. J., Cohen-Kettenis, P., & Melman, T. M. (2001). A randomized controlled trial of risperidone in the treatment of aggression in hospitalized adolescents with subaverage cognitive abilities. *Journal of Clinical Psychiatry, 62*, 239–248.

Findling, R. L., McNamara, N., Branicky, L. A., Schluchter, M. D., Lemon, E., & Blumer, J. L. (2000). A double-blind pilot study of risperidone in the treatment of conduct disorder. *Journal of the American Academy of Child and Adolescent Psychiatry, 39*, 509–516.

Snyder, R., Turgay, A., Aman, M., Binder, C., Fisman, S., Carroll, A., et al. (2002). Effects of risperidone on conduct and disruptive behavior disorders in children with subaverage IQs. *Journal of the American Academy of Child and Adolescent Psychiatry, 41*, 1026–1036.

Van Bellinghen, M., & deTroch, C. (2001). Risperidone in the treatment of behavioral disturbances in children and adolescents with borderline intellectual functioning: A double-blind, placebo-controlled pilot trial. *Journal of Child and Adolescent Psychopharmacology, 11*, 5–13.

Chapter 4

Ensuring the Safety of Children Treated with Second-Generation Antipsychotics

Rebecca Ronsley*, Lorrie Chow†, Kristine Kuss†, Jana Davidson‡,§, Constadina Panagiotopoulos¶,#

*BC Children's Hospital, University of British Columbia, Vancouver, British Columbia, Canada
†Provincial Mental Health Metabolic Program, BC Children's Hospital, Vancouver, British Columbia, Canada
‡Children's & Women's Mental Health and Substance Use Services, Children's and Women's Health Centre of BC, Provincial Health Services Authority, Vancouver, British Columbia, Canada
§Department of Psychiatry, University of British Columbia, Vancouver, British Columbia, Canada
¶BC Children's Hospital, Provincial Health Services Authority, Vancouver, British Columbia, Canada
#Department of Pediatrics, University of British Columbia, Vancouver, British Columbia, Canada

INTRODUCTION

Second-generation antipsychotics (SGAs) are used to treat a wide variety of mental illnesses and symptoms in children and youth (Doey, Handelman, Seabrook, & Steele, 2007; Panagiotopoulos, Ronsley, Elbe, Davidson, & Smith, 2010; Pringsheim, Lam, & Patten, 2011b; Ronsley et al., 2013). Most commonly, they are used to treat insomnia, impulsivity, obsessive-compulsive disorder, post-traumatic stress disorder, and depression (Bachmann, Lempp, Glaeske, & Hoffmann, 2014, pp. 25-34; Domino & Swartz, 2008; Katzmarzyk, 2008; Olfson, Crystal, Huang, & Gerhard, 2010; Ronsley et al. (2013); Panagiotopoulos, Ronsley, & Davidson, 2009; Therapeutics Initiative, 2009). However, the most evidence for their effectiveness in children and youth comes from studies examining SGAs for the treatment of bipolar I disorder, schizophrenia, and disruptive behavior disorders (see Chapter 1 for a summary of clinical trial findings). As a result, Health Canada has approved the SGA aripiprazole for the treatment of schizophrenia in youth aged 15-17 years old and for the treatment of manic or mixed episodes of bipolar I disorder in 13-17 year olds. In contrast, the United States of America Food and Drug Administration (FDA) has approved different SGA drugs for the treatment of schizophrenia, bipolar I disorder, and irritability associated with

The Science and Ethics of Antipsychotic Use in Children. http://dx.doi.org/10.1016/B978-0-12-800016-8.00004-0

TABLE 4.1 FDA-Approved Indications for Second-Generation Antipsychotic use in Children

Antipsychotic	Indication	Target Symptoms	Age Range (Years)
Aripiprazole	Autism	Irritability	6-17
	Bipolar I Disorder	Manic or mixed episodes	10-17
	Schizophrenia		13-17
Olanzapine	Schizophrenia		13-17
	Bipolar I Disorder	Manic or mixed episodes	13-17
Quetiapine	Schizophrenia		13-17
	Bipolar I Disorder	Manic episodes	10-17
Risperidone	Autism	Irritability[a]	5-17
	Bipolar I Disorder	Manic or mixed episodes	10-17
	Schizophrenia		13-17

Note: There are no FDA-approved indications for clozapine or ziprasidone in children.
[a]*Including aggression, temper tantrums, and self-injurious behavior.*

autism in children and youth, which are summarized in (Table 4.1). Despite caution and limited approval by health agencies, SGAs are increasingly being prescribed to Canadian children and youth for nonpsychotic conditions, namely for the treatment of attention-deficit/hyperactivity disorder, mood, anxiety, and conduct disorders, and pervasive developmental disorders (Doey et al., 2007; Pringsheim, Panagiotopoulos, Davidson, Ho, & Canadian Alliance for Monitoring Effectiveness Safety of Antipsychotics in Children (CAMESA) guideline group, 2011). Notably, many of these medications are increasingly being used in the very young (Olfson et al., 2010). A Canadian survey study by Doey et al. (2007) indicated that 12% of all SGA prescriptions were for children 8 years of age and under. In addition, we have accumulated recent data indicating a gender bias in prescribing practices; Canadian boys under the age of 19 are far more likely than girls to receive SGA prescriptions and far more likely to receive prescriptions at a younger age (Ronsley et al., 2013). For instance, rates of prescriptions for boys under 12 years of age are similar to those of teenage girls aged 13-19 years (Panagiotopoulos et al., 2010; Ronsley et al., 2013).

The use of SGAs in children under the age of 12 is especially concerning given our lack of understanding about the long-term effects of antipsychotics on the developing brain and the challenges of making the correct diagnosis for psychiatric problems in the very young. Currently, it is not known whether exposure to antipsychotics in the early years has a harmful or protective influence on brain and central nervous system development; however, research with laboratory animals suggests that some antipsychotic medications may adversely affect the developing brain (Costa, Steardo, & Cuomo, 2004). Moreover, in comparison to adults, the symptom profile of mental health conditions such as schizophrenia and bipolar disorder may vary widely in children and be inconsistent over time (Steele & Fisman, 1997). Long-term studies have shown that the majority of children with mental health problems as toddlers and preschoolers will continue to have a psychiatric diagnosis in their school-age years, though not necessarily for the same condition (Briggs-Gowan & Carter, 2008; Lavigne et al., 1998). Since medications are prescribed to treat specific symptoms or disorders, it is not clear that the medication used for preschool intervention will be the best choice over time (Fanton & Gleason, 2009).

In these instances, it is especially important that a thorough clinical evaluation be completed prior to confirming diagnosis and starting treatment with an antipsychotic. Physicians should always re-examine the primary diagnosis, as a diagnostic error could result in unnecessary or inappropriate use of medications that pose risks for adverse events. Currently, there are many tools available for physicians to assist in the accurate diagnosis of several mental health conditions in children, including attention-deficit/hyperactivity disorder and autism spectrum disorder. In addition, there are diagnostic tools and resources designed to aid primary care physicians in making accurate psychiatric diagnoses (see Appendix A for a list of resources). Referral to a specialist for diagnostic clarification of moderate to severe mental health disorders is generally appropriate. Specifically, disorders such as autism spectrum disorder, bipolar disorder, and psychotic disorders should involve a referral to a child psychiatrist or pediatrician with additional training in developmental or mental health concerns whenever possible. Finally, once treatment with an antipsychotic medication has begun, physicians should monitor the health of children and youth to proactively prevent or manage negative side effects. In this chapter, we focus our discussion on this latter point. We aim to inform the reader about the possible negative side effects associated with SGA use in children and youth and provide recommendations for physicians and families on best practices for medical care and follow-up for young people receiving SGA treatment.

SIDE EFFECTS ASSOCIATED WITH SGA USE IN CHILDREN AND YOUTH

The increase in SGA use has been in part due to the perception that this newer class of drugs is safer. Research suggests that in comparison to older, first-generation drugs, SGAs are associated with fewer or less severe negative side effects, particularly with respect to tardive dyskinesia (involuntary, repetitive body movements) and extrapyramidal side effects such as tremor, slurred speech, akathisia, dystonia, and bradyphrenia (Correll, Leucht, & Kane, 2004;

Kane, 2001). However, recent studies suggest that SGAs are not entirely safe in that they confer greater risk for metabolic adverse events than was previously seen with first-generation antipsychotics. In adults, there is a large body of literature raising concerns about the safety of SGAs with regard to metabolic side effects, which include rapid weight gain, dyslipidemia (abnormal amount of lipids, such as cholesterol or fat, in the blood), insulin resistance, and metabolic syndrome (Cohen, 2004; Henderson, 2007; Meyer & Koro, 2004; Nasrallah, 2008; Nasrallah & Newcomer, 2004; Newcomer et al., 2009; Tandon & Halbreich, 2003; Wu et al., 2006). Metabolic syndrome refers to a cluster of conditions— hypertension, hyperglycemia, central adiposity, and dyslipidemia— that occur together, increasing the risk of heart disease, stroke, and diabetes. In children and adolescents treated with SGAs, there is a growing body of evidence indicating that they are also at risk for central obesity, impaired glucose tolerance, dyslipidemia, hypertension, and metabolic syndrome (Correll, 2005; Correll, Frederickson, Kane, & Manu, 2006; Correll et al., 2009; Panagiotopoulos, Ronsley, Kuzeljevic, & Davidson, 2012; Panagiotopoulos et al., 2009). Furthermore, there is evidence that these metabolic complications may affect children and adolescents to an even greater degree than they affect adults (Correll et al., 2009). In fact, in the first large-scale, prospective cohort study of children, Correll et al. (2009) demonstrated that SGA treatment for an average of 10.8 weeks significantly increased weight gain and body mass index BMI, as well as waist circumference and triglyceride levels in the blood which can lead to atherosclerotic changes and subsequent heart disease. Our work (Panagiotopoulos et al., 2009) supports these findings and has shown that SGA treatment in children is associated with a twofold increased rate of obesity and a threefold increased rate of impaired fasting glucose, which is a precursor to diabetes. Following this study, we conducted a prospective cohort study that demonstrated the presence of metabolic syndrome in 19% of SGA-treated children compared to 0.8% in antipsychotic-naive children, a 30-fold increased odds ratio (Panagiotopoulos et al., 2012). Furthermore, we found an increased prevalence of symptoms associated with impaired metabolic functioning in SGA-treated children compared to controls, such as elevated waist circumference (40.7% in SGA-treated youth vs 10.1% in controls), hypertriglyceridemia (33.7% vs 18.8%), impaired fasting glucose (12.5% vs 0.7%), and hypertension (41.2% vs 16.5%) (Panagiotopoulos et al., 2012). Most recently, others have shown that new users of antipsychotic medications have a threefold increased risk for developing type 2 diabetes within the first year of treatment, a risk that becomes greater (3.14-fold) in children aged 6-17 years as the dose of antipsychotic medication increases (Bobo et al., 2013).

MONITORING THE HEALTH OF CHILDREN AND YOUTH ON SGAs

Despite our knowledge of these potential negative side effects, medical care and follow-up in the form of metabolic monitoring has historically been very low in this population (Morrato, Druss, et al., 2010, Morrato, Nicol, et al., 2010; Panagiotopoulos et al., 2009). One Canadian study conducted on children admitted to a psychiatric emergency unit revealed that only 39% of children receiving SGA treatment had both height and weight measured during their admission, only 43% had a fasting glucose measured, and 32% had a fasting lipid profile measured (Panagiotopoulos et al., 2009). Numerous additional studies conducted in several countries have demonstrated similarly low monitoring rates (Haupt et al., 2009; Khan, Shaikh, & Ablah, 2010; Morrato et al., 2009, 2011; Morrato, Druss, et al., 2010, Morrato, Nicol, et al., 2010; Reeves et al., 2013; Reeves, Kaldany, Lieberman, & Vyas, 2009). This is of utmost concern given that, if left untreated, these negative side effects can increase the risk for serious cardiovascular complications and mortality in adulthood (Burns, Letuchy, Paulos, & Witt, 2009). Studies have shown that adults with mental illness have 15-25 years of reduced life expectancy. Furthermore, adults with mental illness have a 19% greater mortality rate when compared to the general population. This is likely secondary to the burden of psychiatric illness coupled with side effects related to medications used to treat these illnesses (Casey et al., 2004; Cohn, Prud'homme, Streiner, Kameh, & Remington, 2004). Hence, early screening for metabolic side effects is crucial for ensuring early treatment and potential mitigation of long-term adverse health outcomes from this pharmacological treatment (Meyer et al., 2008). Below, we outline metabolic screening initiatives and provide guidance for healthcare professionals and families on best monitoring practices.

GUIDELINES FOR METABOLIC MONITORING

Monitoring for metabolic side effects during SGA treatment requires a regular and comprehensive history (including questioning about carbohydrate craving, polyuria, and polydipsia) and physical exam in addition to laboratory testing, given that metabolic dysregulation in children may not always be readily apparent. In 2004, a joint consensus statement was published by four leading health organizations in the United States (American Diabetes Association, American Psychiatric Association, American Association of Clinical Endocrinologists, & North American Association for the Study of Obesity, 2004) proposing a metabolic monitoring protocol involving regular height, weight, and blood pressure measurements and blood work (including fasting glucose and lipid profile) for SGA-treated adults. After this consensus statement was published, there was a documented improvement in the use of metabolic monitoring for adults, from 1.2% being monitored prior to the release of the protocol to 7.2% after (Morrato et al., 2009).

In 2008, we developed a metabolic monitoring tool (MMT) at British Columbia Children's Hospital in Vancouver, Canada, as a collaborative project between a pediatric endocrinologist (Dr. Constadina Panagiotopoulos) and a child psychiatrist (Dr. Jana Davidson) for inpatient use in children treated with SGAs. Our MMT was produced based on a thorough review of the literature and available adult guidelines as well as consultation with several pediatric and psychiatric subspecialists. Since its development, we have worked to refine the MMT and have created a modified version for outpatient use in the community (see Figure 4.1). Our MMT is now endorsed by the Canadian Academy of Child and Adolescent Psychiatry and the Canadian Pediatric Society. In the

METABOLIC ASSESSMENT, SCREENING AND MONITORING TOOL

BC Mental Health & Addiction Services
An Agency of the Provincial Health Services Authority

BC CHILDREN'S HOSPITAL

P1

Client Details

Client Name (last, first):	PHN:	DOB: (dd/mm/yyyy)
Hospital/Clinic ID:	Gender: □ Male □ Female → □ Menstual □ Pre-menstual	Assessment Date: (dd/mm/yyyy)

Target Symptoms

(Check all that apply with respect to starting Second Generation Antipsychotic (SGA))

□ Mania	□ Motor/vocal tic
□ Mood/affect lability	□ Sedation/ Sleep
□ Mood stabilization (Bipolar Disorder)	□ Aggression
□ Oppositionality	□ Augmentation of _____
□ Psychosis	□ Other (list) _____
□ Self-injurious behaviour	

Diagnoses

Axis I Diagnosis (Primary)	Axis I Diagnosis (Comorbid)	Axis II Diagnosis	Axis III (other medical conditions)	Axis IV	Axis 5 (GAF score)

Ethnicity

□ Aboriginal*	□ South Asian* (i.e. Indian/Pakistani)	□ Asian* (i.e. Japanese/Chinese)
□ Mexican/Hispanic*	□ African/Caribbean*	
□ Caucasian	□ Arab (i.e. Saudi Arabian/Egyptian/Iraqi)	* = high risk ethnicity

Risk Factor Evaluation

Family History

	No	Yes	Unknown	1st degree*	2nd degree*
Diabetes		□ Type 1 □ Type 2 □ Gestational			
Hyperlipidemia					
Cardiovascular Disease					
Schizophrenia					
Schizoaffective Disorder					
Psychosis Not Otherwise Specified					
Bipolar Disorder					

*1st degree relative (mother/father/sibling), 2nd degree relative (grandmother/grandfather/cousin/aunt/uncle)

Individual Risk Factors

Smoking	□ No	□ Yes, _____ cigarettes/day
Physical Activity eg. Exercise (walking)	□ No	□ Yes, _____ min/day
Screen Time eg. computers, tv, video games	□ No	□ Yes, _____ min/day
Sugar-sweetened beverages	□ No	□ Yes, _____ cans of pop/day □ Yes, _____ juice boxes/day

FIGURE 4.1   MMT: whole metabolic monitoring tool (CYMHT version). *(SEPARATE FILE)* Reproduced with permission from the authors.

(Continued)

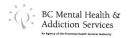

P2

Parameter		Pre-treatment Baseline	1 month	2 month	3 month	6 month	9 month	12 month
Assessment Date (dd/mm/yy): →								
Height (cm)[1]								
Height percentile								
Weight (kg)[1]								
Weight percentile								
BMI: (Wt (kg) / Ht (cm2) x10,000)[1]								
BMI percentile								
Waist Circumference (At the level of the umbilicus)[2]								
Waist Circumference percentile								
Blood Pressure[3] (systolic/diastolic)		/	/	/	/	/	/	/
Blood Pressure percentile (systolic/diastolic)		/	/	/	/	/	/	/
Neurological Examination [4]		☐ completed			☐ completed	☐ completed		☐ completed
Laboratory Evaluations:	Normal Values							
Fasting Plasma Glucose	≤ 6.1 mmol/L[5]							
Fasting Insulin[6]	≤ 100 pmol/L[7]							
Fasting Total Cholesterol	< 5.2 mmol/L							
Fasting LDL-C	< 3.35 mmol/L							
Fasting HDL-C	≥ 1.05 mmol/L							
Fasting Triglycerides	< 1.5 mmol/L							
AST								
ALT								
TSH **(Quetiapine ONLY)**								
Prolactin[8]								
Other_____ (eg. Amylase, A1C, OGTT)[9]								
Physician Initials: →								

Interventions (continue checking as conducted throughout the year)	Pre-treatment	Post-treatment	
	☐ Discuss metabolic risks ☐ Discuss diet ☐ Discuss physical activity ☐ Risk/benefit assessment ☐ Discuss smoking cessation	☐ Discuss diet ☐ Refer to dietitian ☐ Discuss signs and symptoms of diabetes/DKA ☐ Discuss physical activity ☐ Refer to rehab/groups for lifestyle management	☐ Switch antipsychotic medication ☐ Refer to specialized services (via GP) e.g. lipid clinic, diabetes clinic ☐ Liaise with GP re: abnormal labs ☐ Other _____

Comments	
Frequency of follow up after 12 month assessment recommended as yearly or sooner if clinically indicated	

☐ = not recommended

[1] To determine height, weight and BMI percentiles, use age and sex-specific growth charts at: **www.cdc.gov/growthcharts/**
[2] To determine age and sex-specific percentiles, go to: **www.idf.org/webdata/docs/Mets_definition_children.pdf** (pages 18-19)
[3] To determine age and sex-specific percentiles, go to: **www.pediatrics.aappublications.org/cgi/content/full/114/2/S2/555**
[4] Tools available for monitoring extrapyramidal symptoms that may be used: AIMS (Abnormal Involuntary Movement Scale), SAS (Simpson-Angus Scale), ESRS (Extrapyramidal Symptom Rating Scale), BARS (Barnes Akathisia Rating Scale).
[5] For FPG values of 5.6 – 6.0 mmol/L, consideration should be given to performing an oral glucose tolerance test (OGTT)
[6] Note that this assessment is NOT recommended for Aripiprazole or Ziprasidone, but IS appropriate for all other SGAs
[7] For fasting insulin levels > 100 pmol/L, consideration should be given to performing an OGTT
[8] Note that assessment of prolactin levels should be completed according to protocol EXCEPT when the patient is displaying clinical symptoms of hyperprolactinemia (ie: menstrual irregularity, gynecomastia, or galactorrhea), in which case more frequent monitoring may be warranted. Please also note that Risperidone is the SGA with the greatest effect on prolactin
[9] It is recommended that Amylase levels be monitored in cases where the patient presents with clinical symptoms of pancreatitis (ie: abdominal pain, nausea, vomiting)

FIGURE 4.1, CONT'D

tool, we provide detailed checklists for completing anthropometric measurements (weight, height, waist circumference, and blood pressure) and for the monitoring of various blood work parameters (fasting glucose, insulin, fasting lipids, alanine aminotransferase (ALT), aspartate aminotransferase (AST), thyroid stimulating hormone (TSH), and prolactin) at regular time intervals

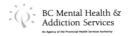

P3

	Drug Initiation	1 month	2 month	3 month	6 month	9 month	12 month
SGAs Assessment Date (dd/mm/yyyy): →							
Risperidone (Risperdal)	Dose ____ Freq ____	Dose ____ Freq ____	Dose ____ Freq ____	Dose ____ Freq ____	Dose ____ Freq ____	Dose ____ Freq ____	Dose ____ Freq ____
Quetiapine (Seroquel)	Dose ____ Freq ____	Dose ____ Freq ____	Dose ____ Freq ____	Dose ____ Freq ____	Dose ____ Freq ____	Dose ____ Freq ____	Dose ____ Freq ____
Olanzapine (Zyprexa)	Dose ____ Freq ____	Dose ____ Freq ____	Dose ____ Freq ____	Dose ____ Freq ____	Dose ____ Freq ____	Dose ____ Freq ____	Dose ____ Freq ____
Paliperidone (Invega)	Dose ____ Freq ____	Dose ____ Freq ____	Dose ____ Freq ____	Dose ____ Freq ____	Dose ____ Freq ____	Dose ____ Freq ____	Dose ____ Freq ____
Clozapine (Clozaril)	Dose ____ Freq ____	Dose ____ Freq ____	Dose ____ Freq ____	Dose ____ Freq ____	Dose ____ Freq ____	Dose ____ Freq ____	Dose ____ Freq ____
Ziprasidone (Zeldox)	Dose ____ Freq ____	Dose ____ Freq ____	Dose ____ Freq ____	Dose ____ Freq ____	Dose ____ Freq ____	Dose ____ Freq ____	Dose ____ Freq ____
Aripiprazole (Abilify)	Dose ____ Freq ____	Dose ____ Freq ____	Dose ____ Freq ____	Dose ____ Freq ____	Dose ____ Freq ____	Dose ____ Freq ____	Dose ____ Freq ____
Other Medications Assessment Date (dd/mm/yyyy): →							
	Dose ____ Freq ____	Dose ____ Freq ____	Dose ____ Freq ____	Dose ____ Freq ____	Dose ____ Freq ____	Dose ____ Freq ____	Dose ____ Freq ____
	Dose ____ Freq ____	Dose ____ Freq ____	Dose ____ Freq ____	Dose ____ Freq ____	Dose ____ Freq ____	Dose ____ Freq ____	Dose ____ Freq ____
	Dose ____ Freq ____	Dose ____ Freq ____	Dose ____ Freq ____	Dose ____ Freq ____	Dose ____ Freq ____	Dose ____ Freq ____	Dose ____ Freq ____
	Dose ____ Freq ____	Dose ____ Freq ____	Dose ____ Freq ____	Dose ____ Freq ____	Dose ____ Freq ____	Dose ____ Freq ____	Dose ____ Freq ____
	Dose ____ Freq ____	Dose ____ Freq ____	Dose ____ Freq ____	Dose ____ Freq ____	Dose ____ Freq ____	Dose ____ Freq ____	Dose ____ Freq ____
	Dose ____ Freq ____	Dose ____ Freq ____	Dose ____ Freq ____	Dose ____ Freq ____	Dose ____ Freq ____	Dose ____ Freq ____	Dose ____ Freq ____
	Dose ____ Freq ____	Dose ____ Freq ____	Dose ____ Freq ____	Dose ____ Freq ____	Dose ____ Freq ____	Dose ____ Freq ____	Dose ____ Freq ____
	Dose ____ Freq ____	Dose ____ Freq ____	Dose ____ Freq ____	Dose ____ Freq ____	Dose ____ Freq ____	Dose ____ Freq ____	Dose ____ Freq ____
Physician Initials: →							
Comments and description of changes made to medication dose at other time interval							
Additional Comments							

Medications

FIGURE 4.1, CONT'D

throughout the first year of SGA treatment, and yearly thereafter. Following the work described above, we joined the Canadian Alliance for Monitoring Effectiveness and Safety of Antipsychotics in Children (CAMESA) to create the first national evidence-based set of guidelines published in Canada (Pringsheim, Panagiotopoulos, Davidson, Ho, and Canadian Alliance for Monitoring Effectiveness Safety of Antipsychotics in Children (CAMESA) guideline group, 2011a). The CAMESA guideline group includes specialists in pediatric neurology, child psychiatry, pediatric endocrinology, and pediatric cardiology as well as a family physician and a pharmacist. These guidelines were developed for use in children 18 years of age and under and were based on a systematic review of the literature. In addition to presenting recommendations for the monitoring of metabolic and neurologic side effects during SGA treatment, the CAMESA guidelines provide the levels of evidence associated with the specific side effects for each antipsychotic medication (see Appendix A for a link to this resource).

Other similar metabolic monitoring guidelines have been developed worldwide for use in SGA-treated children. In the United States, Correll (2008b) published recommendations for regular monitoring of fasting glucose, lipids, TSH, prolactin, and anthropometric measurements with the addition of assessments for sexual and reproductive functioning at 3-month intervals. Furthermore, these guidelines include a discussion of the importance of including patient families in lifestyle modifications surrounding healthy eating and physical activity to reduce weight gain and manage metabolic side effects (Correll, 2008b). In the United Kingdom, one set of guidelines was recently published (Haddad et al., 2013). Haddad et al. (2013) published the *SMARTS* (Systematic Monitoring of Adverse events Related to TreatmentS) checklist. Similar to the MMT we present in Figure 4.1, these guidelines were developed as an interprofessional collaborative project that included psychiatrists, general physicians, and a psychopharmacologist. Although the SMARTS checklist assesses similar metabolic parameters to the previously discussed monitoring protocols, it is designed to be completed by the patient or patient's family rather than the treating physician.

RECOMMENDATIONS FOR MONITORING METABOLIC CHANGES

A holistic approach that includes collaboration with allied health professionals, parent education, and family engagement in lifestyle modification along with regular assessment of metabolic parameters is critical for safeguarding the health of children and youth on SGAs. In Table 4.2, we present a summary of our recommendations for metabolic monitoring at specific time intervals. Below, we provide a general set of guidelines for the types of measurements and medical tools required to ensure consistent and effective monitoring.

Height

Height is best measured using a calibrated stadiometer with an average of two to three measurements. The child should first be instructed to remove his or her shoes and any headwear and be positioned such that the heels are to the back of the stadiometer and the chin is parallel to the floor. See Appendix A for a link to download detailed instructions for accurate measurement of height in children.

TABLE 4.2 Metabolic Monitoring Protocol by Time Interval for Use in Children Treated With Second-Generation Antipsychotics

Clinical Evaluation

	Tools	Baseline	1 month	2 months	3 months	6 months	9 months	12 months
Family and personal history[a]		X						
Height, weight and BMI	www.cdc.gov/growthcharts/	X	X	X	X	X	X	X
Waist circumference	www.idf.org/webdata/docs/Mets_definition_children.pdf	X	X	X	X	X	X	X
Blood pressure	http://keltymentalhealth.ca/sites/default/files/HighBPGuidelines.pdf	X	X	X	X	X	X	X
Neurological examination	• AIMS (Abnormal Involuntary Movement Scale) www.mhsip.org/libarary/pdfFiles/abnormalinvoluntarymovementscale.pdf • SAS (Simpson-Angus Scale) www.outcometracker.org/library/SAS.pdf • ESR (Barnes Akathisia Rating Scale) http://keltymentalhealth.ca/sites/default/files/BARS.pdf	X			X	X		X

TABLE 4.2 Metabolic Monitoring Protocol by Time Interval for Use in Children Treated With Second-Generation Antipsychotics — Cont'd

Laboratory Investigations

	Baseline	1 month	2 months	3 months	6 months	9 months	12 months
Fasting plasma glucose	X			X	X	X	X
Fasting insulin	X			X	X	X	X
Lipid profile (total cholesterol, HDL, LDL, triglycerides)	X			X	X	X	X
AST and ALT	X				X		X
TSH (Quetiapine only)	X						X
Prolactin[b]							X

[a]Family history of diabetes (type 1, type 2, gestational), hyperlipidemia, cardiovascular disease, schizophrenia, schizoaffective disorder, psychosis not otherwise specified, or bipolar disorder; personal history of smoking, physical activity, screen time, and sugar-sweetened beverages.
[b]Assessment of prolactin levels should be completed according to protocol except when the patient displays clinical symptoms of hyperprolactinemia (menstrual irregularity, gynecomastia, or galactorrhea), in which case more frequent monitoring is warranted.
Adapted from the Metabolic Assessment, Screening and Monitoring Tool. Reproduced with permission from original article, Horn et al., BCMJ.

Weight

Weight is best measured using the same digital scale at each appointment. The child should first be instructed to remove heavy outerwear and shoes. Weight is best obtained as an average of two measurements.

Body Mass Index

BMI is calculated as weight (kg)/(height (meters))^2. In children, it is important to assess overweight and obesity status using BMI percentiles for the child's age and sex. BMI percentile calculations and charts are available at the Center for Disease Control website and at the World Health Organization website (see Appendix A for links). "Overweight" is defined as BMI ≥85th percentile and "obese" is defined as BMI ≥95th percentile (Barlow, 2007).

Waist Circumference

To accurately assess central obesity, it is crucial that waist circumference be measured in a consistent manner at each visit. A flexible tape measure should be used. For this reason, we recommend measuring waist circumference at the child's umbilicus. The child should first be instructed to remove heavy clothing. Ensure that the tape measure is parallel to the floor around the child's waist at the level of the umbilicus. An average of two measurements should be used to determine the waist circumference.

Blood Pressure

Blood pressure should be measured when the child is seated comfortably and quietly with an empty bladder. It is important that an appropriate size blood pressure cuff be used. The blood pressure cuff should measure two-thirds of the upper arm and should easily span the circumference of the arm, such that the circumference of the arm is less than two-thirds the length of the cuff. An average of two measurements should be used to assess blood pressure. In children, it is important to assess pre-hypertension and hypertension using blood pressure percentiles that take into account the child's height, age, and sex. These percentiles can be found at the Center for Disease Control website (see Appendix A). "Pre-hypertension" is classified as ≥90th percentile and "hypertension" is classified as ≥95th percentile (Falkner, 2004).

MANAGEMENT OF METABOLIC COMPLICATIONS

Early identification and treatment of metabolic side effects is crucial in mitigating long-term morbidity in children treated with SGAs. Table 4.3 depicts a reference guide for physicians for identification and interpretation of physical exam and laboratory abnormalities and initial management for each as it occurs. The CAMESA guideline for management of side effects describes an approach

TABLE 4.3 Quick Reference Guide for Physicians

Body Mass Index (BMI)

NORMAL BMI	OVERWEIGHT BMI	OBESE BMI
(5th to 85th percentile)	(≥85th and <95th percentile)	(≥95th percentile)
Repeat BMI measurement at next scheduled screen	Re-evaluate use of SGAs to minimize weight	Re-evaluate use of SGAs to minimize weight
	Consider lifestyle intervention aimed at weight loss	Consider lifestyle intervention aimed at weight loss
		Consider metformin in consultation with a specialist

Waist Circumference (WC)

NORMAL	ABDOMINALLY OVERWEIGHT	ABDOMINALLY OBESE
(5th to 75th percentile)	(≥75th and <90th percentile)	(≥90th percentile)
Repeat waist circumference measurement at next scheduled screen	Re-evaluate use of SGAs to minimize weight	Re-evaluate use of SGAs to minimize weight
	Consider lifestyle intervention aimed at weight loss	Consider lifestyle intervention aimed at weight loss
		Consider metformin in consultation with a specialist

Blood Pressure (BP)

NORMAL	PRE-HYPERTENSION	STAGE 1 HYPERTENSION
(SPB and DPB <90th percentile)	(SBP or DPB ≥90th and <95th percentile OR BP exceeds 120/80 mmHg)	(SBP and/or DPB 95th to 99th percentile + 5 mmHg)
Repeat BP check at next scheduled screen	Recheck BP reading in 6 months; if still elevated, consider specialist consultation	Recheck BP reading in 1-2 weeks or sooner if symptomatic
		If persistently elevated on 2 additional occasions, consider specialist consultation for evaluation and treatment within 1 month

(Continued)

TABLE 4.3 Quick Reference Guide for Physicians—cont'd

Body Mass Index (BMI)

STAGE 2 HYPERTENSION	SEVERE HYPERTENSION	
(SBP and/or DBP >99th percentile + 5 mmHg)	(SBP or DBP >95th percentile + >20 mmHg or symptomatic)	
Consult specialist within 1 week, or immediately if patient is symptomatic	Immediate assessment by specialist for investigation and management	
	Patients with symptomatic malignant hypertension should be referred to the nearest emergency room	

Fasting Plasma Glucose (FPG) and Insulin

NORMAL	IMPAIRED	ABNORMAL
(FPG <6.1 mmol/L)	(FPG 6.1-6.9 mmol/L)	(FPG ≥ 7 mmol/L)
Repeat FBP at next scheduled screen	Consider OGTT and specialist consultation if abnormal	Consult with specialist for the management of diabetes
If fasting insulin is above the upper limit of normal for the assay being used, consider OGTT and specialist consultation	Consider metformin in consultation with a specialist	
For an FPG value of 5.6-6.0 mmol/L consideration should be given to an OGTT		

to addressing metabolic complications with SGA treatment (Pringsheim, Panagiotopoulos, Davidson, Ho, & Canadian Alliance for Monitoring Effectiveness Safety of Antipsychotics in Children (CAMESA) guideline group, 2011). Treatment of metabolic side effects should include the following.

1. *Use of lowest effective dose of second-generation antipsychotic medication*: Studies have demonstrated that the risk of metabolic side effects increases with higher SGA doses (Bobo et al., 2013). It is recommended that children always be treated with the lowest dosage of medication that is effective in addressing the symptoms of their mental health condition. The medication dosage should be evaluated regularly and as a first-line mechanism for addressing metabolic adverse events.

2. *Switching to a lower-risk antipsychotic agent*: Studies clearly show that some antipsychotics pose a greater risk for certain metabolic complications than other antipsychotic medications (Correll, 2009). As first-line management for metabolic adverse events, switching to a lower-risk agent should be considered.

3. *Regular physical activity*: Lifestyle modification aimed at increasing physical activity may be effective in reducing weight gain and improving other metabolic side effects associated with second-generation antipsychotic use. Current physical activity recommendations are for children to engage in 60 minutes of moderate to vigorous intensity physical activity daily (see Appendix A for links to guidelines). This should be especially encouraged in children treated with SGAs to help mitigate weight gain and metabolic dysregulation. Healthy lifestyle habits and goals should be discussed at each visit. It is important to inquire about the child's current type, level, and frequency of activity as well as sedentary behavior, including screen time. Motivating children and families to increase physical activity can be challenging. In children with mental illness, motivation for these lifestyle modifications can be further reduced; thus, children treated with SGAs will require additional support to make these changes (Chovil & Panagiotopoulos, 2010). Lifestyle modification should be a collaborative effort between the physician, allied health professionals (when available), the patient, and the family to ensure that realistic goals are set in place. This may include a variety of activities and should be geared toward the child's interests and developmental level. Incorporating physical activity into the child's daily life is often most effective for increasing overall physical activity. Furthermore, it is often helpful to provide information about local recreation facilities and programs when possible to encourage exploration of a variety of activities. Finally, it may be helpful to provide families with available handouts and websites with strategies for incorporating physical activity into their child's life. This will reinforce the information presented in the office and provide additional resources for the family to learn further strategies. A patient and family tip sheet for increasing physical activity is presented in Table 4.4.

4. *Diet modification*: Children treated with SGA medications often experience cravings for high fat and high carbohydrate foods (Cuerda, Velasco, Merchan-Naranjo, Garcia-Peris, & Arango, 2014). A variety of dietary intervention strategies have been explored in antipsychotic-treated patients. These include food diaries, education surrounding dietary habits, goal setting strategies for diet modification, reduction in total caloric intake, stimulus control, and motivational counseling (Alvarez-Jimenez, Hetrick, Gonzalez-Blanch, Gleeson, & McGorry, 2008; Alvarez-Jimenez et al., 2006; Attux et al., 2011, 2013; Brar et al., 2005; Evans, Newton, & Higgins, 2005; Littrell, Hilligoss, Kirshner, Petty, & Johnson, 2003; Menza et al., 2004; Scocco, Longo, & Caon, 2006; Weber & Wyne, 2006). Currently, it is recommended that strategies for diet modification in children treated with SGAs involve a collaborative effort between the patient, the patient's family, and the healthcare team and include one or all of the following, depending on the needs of the family: (1) self-monitoring of behavior (through food diaries); (2) assessment of motivation and motivational counseling; (3) stimulus control (e.g., utilizing mindful eating, keeping highly palatable foods out

TABLE 4.4 QuickTips for Children and Families

Physical Activity	Nutrition
Spend 60 min being physically active each day (moderate to vigorous intensity)	Increase water-based foods before meals to fill up stomach and decrease portions (e.g., broth-based vegetable soup, water, milk, raw vegetables)
Add active transport to your day (walking, biking, scootering to school, friend's house, etc.)	Increase fiber—slowly work up from 2 g/serving to >4 g per serving; keep sugar to <10 g per serving with cereals, granola bars, etc.
Decrease sedentary time after school by setting a schedule (chores, homework, physical activity) or going to a park or recreation centre	Eat regular meals and snacks to prevent the body from getting overly hungry, which causes overeating; make sure to eat breakfast every day
Try new activities together as a family	Eat out less than once per week
Find an activity that you enjoy—you are much more likely to continue with it	Limit foods that cause weight gain and overeating; keep chips, soda, and processed meats out of the house
Set limits on recreational screen time—maximum 2 h per day; no screens in child's bedroom	Eat mindfully to prevent overeating; don't eat in front of the TV, while playing video games, or while driving
Find ways to overcome barriers to activity; start small and build up activity slowly for better compliance	Stay away from sugar-sweetened beverages such as pop, energy drinks, frapuccinos, sports drinks, iced tea

of sight); (4) education on nutrition principles (e.g., food groups and appropriate portions); and goal setting. These strategies, in conjunction with family education surrounding recommended food group and caloric intake and motivational counseling as well as collaboration with the patient's family to plan realistic goals, are recommended for addressing metabolic side effects during SGA treatment. A patient and family tip sheet for dietary modification during SGA treatment is presented in Table 4.4. Recommended food group and caloric intakes can be found on the Canada Food Guide Health Canada website, and recommendations for appropriate portions can be found on the Canadian Diabetes Association website (see Appendix A for links).

5. *Reduction in polypharmacy*: Recent literature has shown that the concurrent use of multiple psychotropic medications, also known as *polypharmacy*, is associated with increased metabolic and cardiovascular adverse outcomes in children (Correll, 2009). It is important that, whenever possible, polypharmacy is reduced to the use of one antipsychotic medication when treating children with mental health conditions.

TABLE 4.5 Resources for Promoting Healthy Living and Addressing Metabolic Side Effects in Second-Generation Antipsychotic-Treated Children

Resource	Website
Kelty Mental Health Resource Center—provides many healthy living resources for children with mental health conditions, including healthy living toolkits containing specific strategies to help mitigate metabolic side effects during second-generation antipsychotic treatment	http://keltymentalhealth.ca/toolkits/ http://keltymentalhealth.ca/metabolic
British Columbia Mental Health & Substance Use Services Metabolic Program—provides many resources for physicians, including current literature, handbooks, and guidelines for monitoring metabolic side effects in second-generation antipsychotic-treated patients and toolkits for families describing presentation and treatment of side effects during antipsychotic treatment	http://www.bcmhsus.ca/resources/metabolic-program
Public Health Agency of Canada—provides healthy living resources for Canadians of all ages	www.phac-aspc.gc.ca/hp-ps/hl-mvs/index-eng.php
The General Practice Services Committee—provides healthy living resources for Canadians with mental health conditions	www.gpscbc.ca/psp-learning/mental-health/tools-resources

There are many resource available that can help with promoting healthy living and addressing metabolic side effects in antipsychotic-treated children (Table 4.5).

WHY STANDARDIZED METABOLIC MONITORING MATTERS

Improving Patient Care

The use of standardized metabolic monitoring protocols has been shown to significantly improve monitoring rates both in Canada and worldwide (Khan et al., 2010; Mitchell, Delaffon, Vancampfort, Correll, & De Hert, 2012; Ronsley, Rayter, Smith, Davidson, & Panagiotopoulos, 2012). For instance, within an inpatient setting at BC Children's Hospital, the use of the MMT resulted in a dramatic increase in the number of assessments for height (from 39% to 89%), lipid profiles (from 32% to 89%), and fasting glucose measurements (from 34%

to 89%) (Panagiotopoulos et al., 2012). Similarly, when our modified outpatient version of the MMT was applied in community clinics, metabolic monitoring rates for all recommended parameters increased significantly: weight measurements increased from 18.1% at baseline to 51.9%; height measurements increased from 13.5% to 43.2%; waist circumference measurements increased from 2.3% to 21.0%; blood pressure measurements increased from 9.4% to 33.3%; fasting glucose measurements increased from 13.5% to 49.4%; and lipid measurements increased from 11.7% to 49.4% (Ronsley et al., 2012). Rates of metabolic monitoring in SGA-treated children and youth have continued to rise since initial evaluation of this protocol.

Educating Families

Active family engagement is a vital component of successful care of children (Chovil & Panagiotopoulos, 2010). Patients' families serve as key partners not only in the prevention but also in the identification and management of metabolic adverse events during SGA treatment. During focus groups, parents of SGA-treated children expressed interest in understanding potential adverse events with treatment and were keen to learn how to identify concerning changes in their children (Chovil & Panagiotopoulos, 2010). At the initiation of antipsychotic treatment, it is strongly recommended that patients and families receive counseling concerning nutrition, exercise, and healthy lifestyle, regardless of the patient's baseline BMI (Correll, 2008a,2008b; Ho et al., 2011). In fact, parents of children treated with SGAs stated in focus groups that it would be easier to promote good nutrition at the beginning of treatment rather than waiting until weight gain had occurred (Chovil & Panagiotopoulos, 2010). By educating families on good nutrition and physical activity strategies at the beginning of treatment, they serve as partners in the child's health and may mitigate the onset of weight gain and metabolic disruptions.

OVERCOMING BARRIERS TO COMPLETION OF MONITORING

Despite improvements in metabolic monitoring following the creation and use of standardized protocols (Dhamane, Martin, Brixner, Hudson, & Said, 2013; Panagiotopoulos et al., 2009), monitoring remains a problem with some patients. Many groups have identified barriers to the completion of proper metabolic monitoring (see Table 4.6 for details). Commonly identified barriers include lack of proper equipment for anthropometric measurements in community offices, lack of clinician confidence in proper measurement techniques, discontinuity in care when a child is transferred to a new clinical setting, lack of clinical knowledge about the timing and choice of laboratory tests, physician forgetfulness about schedule for metabolic monitoring parameters, and patient needle phobia (Chovil & Panagiotopoulos, 2010; Mangurian et al., 2013; Ronsley, Raghuram, Davidson, & Panagiotopoulos, 2011).

TABLE 4.6 Barriers and Facilitators to Metabolic Monitoring in SGA-Treated Children

Barrier	Strategy
Patient and Family Factors	
Needle Phobia	• Educate children about venipuncture procedure using visuals and dolls to demonstrate
Reduction in adherence to medication with addition of metabolic monitoring	• Provide families with resources explaining antipsychotic treatment and indications for metabolic monitoring as well as identification and treatment of potential side effects • Provide adolescents with age-specific resources about their medication, their potential benefits and potential risks
Healthcare Provider Factors	
Lack of equipment for anthropometric measurements	• Provide healthcare teams with standard equipment lists for each site. Equipment should be comparable to nearby mental health teams and partnering hospital to ensure consistency of monitoring during transfer of care
Lack of clinician confidence in anthropometric measurements	• At implementation of standardized measurement protocol, include in-person training for all clinicians in completing each anthropometric measurement
Inconsistent timing of laboratory investigations	• Use preprinted order sets for each time point to ensure that metabolic laboratory parameters are not missed
Lack of clinician confidence in interpretation of laboratory results	• Provide physicians and allied health care professionals with electronic and paper resources. A currently available handbook includes anthropometric measurements and pediatric norms as well as clinical information about screening for and diagnosing diabetes and metabolic syndrome
Physician forgetfulness with metabolic monitoring parameter timing	• Use a standardized reminder system for all patients to assist physicians in identifying each time point and appropriate investigations

To address concerns with availability of equipment in the community, it is recommended that teams be provided with standard equipment lists that include equipment used by nearby mental health teams and partnering hospitals to ensure continuity and consistency with monitoring if a child's care is transferred. In fact, in one study that assessed effectiveness of site-wide implementation of an MMT in community child and youth mental health teams, assistance was provided with identifying and purchasing appropriate measurement equipment and setting up examination rooms at each site (Ronsley et al., 2011) prior to metabolic monitoring protocol implementation.

To assist healthcare professionals to gain confidence in conducting metabolic monitoring and to ensure consistency between healthcare settings, we recommend that all physicians and allied health professionals receive in-person hands-on training for each of the anthropometric measurements at the time of implementation of a standardized measurement protocol. In addition, given that many clinicians have expressed concern about remembering which laboratory tests to order at each time interval, we suggest using preprinted order sheets to help ensure that metabolic lab parameters are not missed, thus avoiding additional needle pokes for children. Our work has shown that preprinted order sheets reduce the amount of time needed to complete monitoring and the number of instances that children returned to the laboratory for additional blood tests due to missed orders (Ronsley et al., 2011). Furthermore, to address clinician concern about the ability to interpret laboratory investigations and organize appropriate follow-up (Ronsley et al., 2011), we provide electronic and paper references for metabolic monitoring in youth. To do this efficiently, we have created a clinician handbook that includes blood pressure, waist circumference, and BMI norms for the pediatric population, as well as clinical information about screening and the diagnostic criteria for diabetes and metabolic syndrome. See Appendix A for a web link to download a copy of our handbook.

Finally, physicians regularly report that it is difficult to keep track of each metabolic monitoring time point for each of their patients. To address this, we recommend that a reminder system be implemented in each clinical setting to assist physicians with identifying the recommended investigations for each time point. For the previously mentioned community mental health teams, we sent reminders to physicians 2 weeks before each time point for each patient, which greatly helped assure that monitoring was completed on time (Ronsley et al., 2011).

There are also patient and family factors that may serve as barriers to completing metabolic monitoring. One commonly described barrier is the child's needle phobia (Chovil & Panagiotopoulos, 2010). It is recommended that children be educated at a developmentally appropriate level on the procedure for venipuncture. Previous studies have shown that the use of visuals and/or dolls to demonstrate the venipuncture can significantly relieve anxiety and promote child comfort during this procedure. Finally, it has been reported that families express concern that metabolic monitoring may affect their child's adherence to taking the medication. To help facilitate monitoring, it is recommended that families be provided with resources that explain antipsychotic treatment, metabolic monitoring, and identification and treatment of metabolic side effects. To address this need, a helpful resource from the Kelty Mental Health Resource Centre in British Columbia was recently created regarding patient and family concerns and is available online (see Appendix A for details).

CONCLUSION

Safe use of SGAs in children must be a priority for all prescribers. First and foremost, this starts with ensuring that these medications are used for evidence-based indications, and that regular monitoring for metabolic side effects occurs at baseline and regular intervals thereafter per recommended guidelines. It is crucial that physicians as well as allied healthcare professionals receive training regarding the procedures and protocols for metabolic monitoring, as well as the tools required to identify and manage metabolic complications during SGA treatment. Finally, it is important to engage parents and caregivers to support children with proactive lifestyle modification to prevent and treat the potential adverse metabolic side effects associated with these medications. There are many resources available to assist physicians and other mental health professionals in preventing and treating metabolic side effects in SGA-treated children. For a complete list of resources, see Appendix A.

REFERENCES

Alvarez-Jimenez, M., Gonzalez-Blanch, C., Vazquez-Barquero, J. L., Perez-Iglesias, R., Martinez-Garcia, O., Perez-Pardal, T., et al. (2006). Attenuation of antipsychotic-induced weight gain with early behavioral intervention in drug-naive first-episode psychosis patients: A randomized controlled trial. *The Journal of Clinical Psychiatry, 67*(8), 1253–1260.

Alvarez-Jimenez, M., Hetrick, S. E., Gonzalez-Blanch, C., Gleeson, J. F., & McGorry, P. D. (2008). Non-pharmacological management of antipsychotic-induced weight gain: Systematic review and meta-analysis of randomised controlled trials. *The British Journal of Psychiatry: the Journal of Mental Science, 193*(2), 101–107. http://dx.doi.org/10.1192/bjp.bp.107.042853.

American Diabetes Association, American Psychiatric Association, American Association of Clinical Endocrinologists, & North American Association for the Study of Obesity. (2004). Consensus development conference on antipsychotic drugs and obesity and diabetes. *Diabetes Care, 27*(2), 596–601.

Attux, C., Martini, L. C., Araujo, C. M., Roma, A. M., Reis, A. F., & Bressan, R. A. (2011). The effectiveness of a non-pharmacological intervention for weight gain management in severe mental disorders: Results from a national multicentric study. *Revista Brasileira De Psiquiatria (Sao Paulo, Brazil: 1999), 33*(2), 117–121.

Attux, C., Martini, L. C., Elkis, H., Tamai, S., Freirias, A., Md, Camargo, et al. (2013). A 6-month randomized controlled trial to test the efficacy of a lifestyle intervention for weight gain management in schizophrenia. *BMC Psychiatry, 13*, 60.

Bachmann, C. J., Lempp, T. F., Glaeske, G. F., & Hoffmann, F. (2014). Antipsychotic prescription in children and adolescents: An analysis of data from a german statutory health insurance company from 2005 to 2012. *Deutsches Ärzteblatt International, 111*(3), 25–34.

Barlow, S. E. (2007). Expert committee recommendations regarding the prevention, assessment, and treatment of child and adolescent overweight and obesity: Summary report. *Pediatrics*, 12(120 Suppl. 4), s164–s192.

Bobo, W., Cooper, W., Stein, C., Olfson, M., Graham, D., Daugherty, J., et al. (2013). Antipsychotics and the risk of type 2 diabetes mellitus in children and youth. *JAMA Psychiatry*, 70(10), 1067–1075.

Brar, J. S., Ganguli, R., Pandina, G., Turkoz, I., Berry, S., & Mahmoud, R. (2005). Effects of behavioral therapy on weight loss in overweight and obese patients with schizophrenia or schizoaffective disorder. *The Journal of Clinical Psychiatry*, 66(2), 205–212.

Briggs-Gowan, M. J., & Carter, A. S. (2008). Social-emotional screening status in early childhood predicts elementary school outcomes. *Pediatrics*, 121(5), 957–962. http://dx.doi.org/10.1542/peds.2007-1948; 10.1542/peds.2007-1948.

Burns, T. L., Letuchy, E. M., Paulos, R., & Witt, J. (2009). Childhood predictors of the metabolic syndrome in middle-aged adults: The muscatine study. *The Journal of Pediatrics*, 155(3), S5. http://dx.doi.org/10.1016/j.jpeds.2009.04.044 e17-26.

Casey, D. E., Haupt, D. W., Newcomer, J. W., Henderson, D. C., Sernyak, M. J., Davidson, M., et al. (2004). Antipsychotic-induced weight gain and metabolic abnormalities: Implications for increased mortality in patients with schizophrenia. *The Journal of Clinical Psychiatry*, 65(Suppl. 7), 4–18; quiz 19–20.

Chovil, N., & Panagiotopoulos, C. (2010). Engaging families in research to determine health literacy needs related to the use of second-generation antipsychotics in children and adolescents. *Journal of the Canadian Academy of Child and Adolescent Psychiatry*, 19(3), 201–208.

Cohen, D. (2004). Atypical antipsychotics and new onset diabetes mellitus. an overview of the literature. *Pharmacopsychiatry*, 37(1), 1–11. http://dx.doi.org/10.1055/s-2004-815468.

Cohn, T., Prud'homme, D., Streiner, D., Kameh, H., & Remington, G. (2004). Characterizing coronary heart disease risk in chronic schizophrenia: High prevalence of the metabolic syndrome. *Canadian Journal of Psychiatry*, 49(11), 753–760.

Correll, C. U. (2005). Metabolic side effects of second-generation antipsychotics in children and adolescents: A different story? *The Journal of Clinical Psychiatry*, 66(10), 1331–1332.

Correll, C. U. (2008a). Antipsychotic use in children and adolescents: Minimizing adverse effects to maximize outcomes. *Journal of the American Academy of Child and Adolescent Psychiatry*, 47(1), 9–20. http://dx.doi.org/10.1097/chi.0b013e31815b5cb1.

Correll, C. U. (2008b). Monitoring and management of antipsychotic-related metabolic and endocrine adverse events in pediatric patients. *International Review of Psychiatry (Abingdon, England)*, 20(2), 195–201. http://dx.doi.org/10.1080/09540260801889179.

Correll, C. U. (2009). Multiple antipsychotic use associated with metabolic and cardiovascular adverse events in children and adolescents. *Evidence-Based Mental Health*, 12(3), 93. http://dx.doi.org/10.1136/ebmh.12.3.93.

Correll, C. U., Frederickson, A. M., Kane, J. M., & Manu, P. (2006). Metabolic syndrome and the risk of coronary heart disease in 367 patients treated with second-generation antipsychotic drugs. *The Journal of Clinical Psychiatry*, 67(4), 575–583.

Correll, C. U., Leucht, S., & Kane, J. M. (2004). Lower risk for tardive dyskinesia associated with second-generation antipsychotics: A systematic review of 1-year studies. *The American Journal of Psychiatry*, 161(3), 414–425.

Correll, C. U., Manu, P., Olshanskiy, V., Napolitano, B., Kane, J. M., & Malhotra, A. K. (2009). Cardiometabolic risk of second-generation antipsychotic medications during first-time use in children and adolescents. *JAMA, the Journal of the American Medical Association*, 302(16), 1765–1773. http://dx.doi.org/10.1001/jama.2009.1549.

Costa, L. G., Steardo, L. F., & Cuomo, V. (2004). Structural effects and neurofunctional sequelae of developmental exposure to psychotherapeutic drugs: Experimental and clinical aspects. *Pharmacological Reviews, 56*(1), 103–147.

Cuerda, C., Velasco, C., Merchan-Naranjo, J., Garcia-Peris, P., & Arango, C. (2014). The effects of second-generation antipsychotics on food intake, resting energy expenditure and physical activity. *European Journal of Clinical Nutrition, 68*(2), 146–152.

Dhamane, A. D., Martin, B. C., Brixner, D. I., Hudson, T. J., & Said, Q. (2013). Metabolic monitoring of patients prescribed second-generation antipsychotics. *Journal of Psychiatric Practice, 19*(5), 360–374. http://dx.doi.org/10.1097/01.pra.0000435035.45308.03; 10.1097/01.pra.0000435035.45308.03.

Doey, T., Handelman, K., Seabrook, J. A., & Steele, M. (2007). Survey of atypical antipsychotic prescribing by canadian child psychiatrists and developmental pediatricians for patients aged under 18 years. *Canadian Journal of Psychiatry, 52*(6), 363–368.

Domino, M. E., & Swartz, M. S. (2008). Who are the new users of antipsychotic medications? *Psychiatric Services (Washington, DC), 59*(5), 507–514. http://dx.doi.org/10.1176/appi. ps.59.5.507.

Evans, S., Newton, R., & Higgins, S. (2005). Nutritional intervention to prevent weight gain in patients commenced on olanzapine: A randomized controlled trial. *The Australian and New Zealand Journal of Psychiatry, 39*(6), 479–486. http://dx.doi.org/10.1111/j.1440-1614.2005.01607.x.

Falkner, B. (2004). National high blood pressure education program working group on high blood pressure in children and adolescents: The fourth report on the diagnosis, evaluation, and treatment of high blood pressure in children and adolescents. *Pediatrics, 114*, 555–576.

Fanton, J., & Gleason, M. M. (2009). Psychopharmacology and preschoolers: A critical review of current conditions. *Child and Adolescent Psychiatric Clinics of North America, 18*(3), 753–771. http://dx.doi.org/10.1016/j.chc.2009.02.005; 10.1016/j.chc.2009.02.005.

Haddad, P. M., Fleischhacker, W. W., Peuskens, J., Cavallaro, R., Lean, M. E., Morozova, M., et al. (2013). SMARTS (systematic monitoring of adverse events related to TreatmentS): The development of a pragmatic patientcompleted checklist to assess antipsychotic drug side effects. *Therapeutic Advances in Psychopharmacology, 4*, 15–21. http://dx.doi. org/10.1177/2045125313510195.

Haupt, D. W., Rosenblatt, L. C., Kim, E., Baker, R. A., Whitehead, R., & Newcomer, J. W. (2009). Prevalence and predictors of lipid and glucose monitoring in commercially insured patients treated with second-generation antipsychotic agents. *The American Journal of Psychiatry, 166*(3), 345–353. http://dx.doi.org/10.1176/appi.ajp.2008.08030383.

Henderson, D. C. (2007). Weight gain with atypical antipsychotics: Evidence and insights. *The Journal of Clinical Psychiatry, 68*(Suppl. 12), 18–26.

Ho, J., Panagiotopoulos, C., McCrindle, B., Grisaru, S., Pringsheim, T., CAMESA guideline group. (2011). Management recommendations for metabolic complications associated with second generation antipsychotic use in children and youth. *Journal of the Canadian Academy of Child and Adolescent Psychiatry, 20*(3), 234–241.

Kane, J. M. (2001). Extrapyramidal side effects are unacceptable. *European Neuropsychopharmacology: The Journal of the European College of Neuropsychopharmacology, 11*(Suppl. 4), S397–S403.

Katzmarzyk, P. T. (2008). Obesity and physical activity among aboriginal canadians. *Obesity (Silver Spring, Md), 16*(1), 184–190. http://dx.doi.org/10.1038/oby.2007.51.

Khan, A. Y., Shaikh, M. R., & Ablah, E. (2010). To examine the extent of compliance to the proposed monitoring protocol among practicing psychiatrists for second generation antipsychotics. *The Journal of the Pakistan Medical Association, 60*(6), 446–450.

Lavigne, J. V., Arend, R., Rosenbaum, D., Binns, H. J., Christoffel, K. K., & Gibbons, R. D. (1998). Psychiatric disorders with onset in the preschool years: I. stability of diagnoses. *Journal of the American Academy of Child and Adolescent Psychiatry, 37*(12), 1246–1254. http://dx.doi. org/10.1097/00004583-199812000-00007.

Littrell, K. H., Hilligoss, N. M., Kirshner, C. D., Petty, R. G., & Johnson, C. G. (2003). The effects of an educational intervention on antipsychotic-induced weight gain. *Journal of Nursing Scholarship, 35*(3), 237–241.

Mangurian, C., Giwa, F., Shumway, M., Fuentes-Afflick, E., Perez-Stable, E. J., Dilley, J. W., et al. (2013). Primary care providers' views on metabolic monitoring of outpatients taking antipsychotic medication. *Psychiatric Services (Washington, DC), 64*(6), 597–599. http:// dx.doi.org/10.1176/appi.ps.002542012; 10.1176/appi.ps.002542012.

Menza, M., Vreeland, B., Minsky, S., Gara, M., Radler, D. R., & Sakowitz, M. (2004). Managing atypical antipsychotic-associated weight gain: 12-month data on a multimodal weight control program. *The Journal of Clinical Psychiatry, 65*(4), 471–477.

Meyer, J. M., Davis, V. G., Goff, D. C., McEvoy, J. P., Nasrallah, H. A., Davis, S. M., et al. (2008). Change in metabolic syndrome parameters with antipsychotic treatment in the CATIE schizophrenia trial: Prospective data from phase 1. *Schizophrenia Research, 101*(1–3), 273–286.

Meyer, J. M., & Koro, C. E. (2004). The effects of antipsychotic therapy on serum lipids: A comprehensive review. *Schizophrenia Research, 70*(1), 1–17. http://dx.doi.org/10.1016/j. schres.2004.01.014.

Mitchell, A. J., Delaffon, V., Vancampfort, D., Correll, C. U., & De Hert, M. (2012). Guideline concordant monitoring of metabolic risk in people treated with antipsychotic medication: Systematic review and meta-analysis of screening practices. *Psychological Medicine, 42*(1), 125–147. http://dx.doi.org/10.1017/S003329171100105X; 10.1017/ S003329171100105X.

Morrato, E. H., Druss, B., Hartung, D. M., Valuck, R. J., Allen, R., Campagna, E., et al. (2010). Metabolic testing rates in 3 state medicaid programs after FDA warnings and ADA/APA recommendations for second-generation antipsychotic drugs. *Archives of General Psychiatry, 67*(1), 17–24. http://dx.doi.org/10.1001/archgenpsychiatry.2009.179.

Morrato, E. H., Druss, B. G., Hartung, D. M., Valuck, R. J., Thomas, D., Allen, R., et al. (2011). Small area variation and geographic and patient-specific determinants of metabolic testing in antipsychotic users. *Pharmacoepidemiology and Drug Safety, 20*(1), 66–75. http://dx.doi. org/10.1002/pds.2062; 10.1002/pds.2062.

Morrato, E. H., Newcomer, J. W., Kamat, S., Baser, O., Harnett, J., & Cuffel, B. (2009). Metabolic screening after the american diabetes association's consensus statement on antipsychotic drugs and diabetes. *Diabetes Care, 32*(6), 1037–1042. http://dx.doi. org/10.2337/dc08-1720.

Morrato, E. H., Nicol, G. E., Maahs, D., Druss, B. G., Hartung, D. M., Valuck, R. J., et al. (2010). Metabolic screening in children receiving antipsychotic drug treatment. *Archives of Pediatrics & Adolescent Medicine, 164*(4), 344–351. http://dx.doi.org/10.1001/archpediatrics.2010.48.

Nasrallah, H. A. (2008). Atypical antipsychotic-induced metabolic side effects: Insights from receptor-binding profiles. *Molecular Psychiatry, 13*(1), 27–35. http://dx.doi.org/10.1038/ sj.mp.4002066.

Nasrallah, H. A., & Newcomer, J. W. (2004). Atypical antipsychotics and metabolic dysregulation: Evaluating the risk/benefit equation and improving the standard of care. *Journal of Clinical Psychopharmacology, 24*(5 Suppl. 1), S7–S14.

Newcomer, J. W., Ratner, R. E., Eriksson, J. W., Emsley, R., Meulien, D., Miller, F., et al. (2009). A 24-week, multicenter, open-label, randomized study to compare changes in glucose metabolism in patients with schizophrenia receiving treatment with olanzapine, quetiapine, or risperidone. *The Journal of Clinical Psychiatry, 70*(4), 487–499.

Olfson, M., Crystal, S., Huang, C., & Gerhard, T. (2010). Trends in antipsychotic drug use by very young, privately insured children. *Journal of the American Academy of Child and Adolescent Psychiatry, 49*(1), 13–23.

Panagiotopoulos, C., Ronsley, R., & Davidson, J. (2009). Increased prevalence of obesity and glucose intolerance in youth treated with second-generation antipsychotic medications. *Canadian Journal of Psychiatry, 54*(11), 743–749.

Panagiotopoulos, C., Ronsley, R., Elbe, D., Davidson, J., & Smith, D. H. (2010). First do no harm: Promoting an evidence-based approach to atypical antipsychotic use in children and adolescents. *Journal of the Canadian Academy of Child and Adolescent Psychiatry, 19*(2), 124–137.

Panagiotopoulos, C., Ronsley, R., Kuzeljevic, B., & Davidson, J. (2012). Waist circumference is a sensitive screening tool for assessment of metabolic syndrome risk in children treated with second-generation antipsychotics. *Canadian Journal of Psychiatry, 57*(1), 34–44.

Pringsheim, T., Lam, D., & Patten, S. B. (2011). The pharmacoepidemiology of antipsychotic medications for canadian children and adolescents: 2005–2009 RID B-4434-2011. *Journal of Child and Adolescent Psychopharmacology, 21*(6), 537–543. http://dx.doi.org/10.1089/cap.2010.0145.

Pringsheim, T., Panagiotopoulos, C., Davidson, J., Ho, J., Canadian Alliance for Monitoring Effectiveness Safety of Antipsychotics in Children (CAMESA) guideline group. (2011). Evidence-based recommendations for monitoring safety of second-generation antipsychotics in children and youth. *Paediatrics & Child Health, 16*(9), 581–589.

Reeves, R., Kaldany, H., Lieberman, J., & Vyas, R. (2009). Creation of a metabolic monitoring program for second-generation (atypical) antipsychotics. *Journal of Correctional Health Care: The Official Journal of the National Commission on Correctional Health Care, 15*(4), 292–301. http://dx.doi.org/10.1177/1078345809340424.

Reeves, G. M., Keeton, C., Correll, C. U., Johnson, J. L., Hamer, R. M., Sikich, L., et al. (2013). Improving metabolic parameters of antipsychotic child treatment (IMPACT) study: Rationale, design, and methods. *Child and Adolescent Psychiatry and Mental Health, 7*(1), 31. http://dx.doi.org/10.1186/1753-2000-7-31; 10.1186/1753-2000-7-31.

Ronsley, R., Raghuram, K., Davidson, J., & Panagiotopoulos, C. (2011). Barriers and facilitators to implementation of a metabolic monitoring protocol in hospital and community settings for second-generation antipsychotic-treated youth. *Journal of the Canadian Academy of Child and Adolescent Psychiatry, 20*(2), 134–141.

Ronsley, R., Rayter, M., Smith, D., Davidson, J., & Panagiotopoulos, C. (2012). Metabolic monitoring training program implementation in the community setting was associated with improved monitoring in second-generation antipsychotic-treated children. *Canadian Journal of Psychiatry, 57*(5), 292–299.

Ronsley, R., Scott, D., Warburton, W. P., Hamdi, R. D., Louie, D. C., Davidson, J., et al. (2013). A population-based study of antipsychotic prescription trends in children and adolescents in british columbia, from 1996 to 2011. *Canadian Journal of Psychiatry, 58*(6), 361–369.

Scocco, P., Longo, R. F., & Caon, F. (2006). Weight change in treatment with olanzapine and a psychoeducational approach. *Eating Behaviors, 7*(2), 115–124.

Steele, M., & Fisman, S. (1997). Bipolar disorder in children and adolescents: Current challenges. *Canadian Journal of Psychiatry, 42*, 632–636.

Tandon, R., & Halbreich, U. (2003). The second-generation 'atypical' antipsychotics: Similar improved efficacy but different neuroendocrine side effects. *Psychoneuroendocrinology, 28*(Suppl. 1), 1–7.

Therapeutics Initiative. (2009). Increasing use of newer antipsychotics in children: A cause for concern? Therapeutics Initiative: Evidence Based Drug Therapy, April-June 2009.

Weber, M., & Wyne, K. (2006). A cognitive/behavioral group intervention for weight loss in patients treated with atypical antipsychotics. *Schizophrenia Research*, *83*(1), 95–101. http://dx.doi.org/10.1016/j.schres.2006.01.008.

Wu, R. R., Zhao, J. P., Liu, Z. N., Zhai, J. G., Guo, X. F., Guo, W. B., et al. (2006). Effects of typical and atypical antipsychotics on glucose-insulin homeostasis and lipid metabolism in first-episode schizophrenia. *Psychopharmacology*, *186*(4), 572–578. http://dx.doi.org/10.1007/s00213-006-0384-5.

Chapter 5

Pediatric Clinical Trial Activity for Antipsychotics and the Sharing of Results: A Complex Ethical Landscape

Edel Mc Glanaghy[*], Nina Di Pietro[*], Benjamin Wilfond[†,‡]

[*]*National Core for Neuroethics, Division of Neurology, Faculty of Medicine, University of British Columbia, Vancouver, British Columbia, Canada*
[†]*Treuman Katz Center for Pediatric Bioethics, Seattle Children's Research Institute, Seattle, Washington, USA*
[‡]*Department of Pediatrics, University of Washington School of Medicine, Seattle, Washington, USA*

INTRODUCTION

It is estimated that 10-20% of children and youth in Canada suffer from mental illness (Canadian Mental Health Association, 2014). Psychiatric conditions can have a devastating effect on a child or adolescent's developmental trajectory, and there is demand for effective interventions. Yet a review of neuropsychiatric research from 2006 to 2010 revealed that only 10% of clinical trials focused on children (Murthy, Mandl, & Bourgeois, 2013). In line with this, there is a recent consensus that more clinical trials are required to assess the safety and efficacy of second-generation antipsychotic medications (APs) for children and adolescents (Canadian Paediatric Society & Drug Therapy and Hazardous Substances Committee, 2011). When considering the use of APs in young people, physicians and families must consider whether the benefits outweigh the risks. These decisions are best informed by clinical trial data. Historically, however, there have been concerns about including children in research because they represent a particularly vulnerable population. Children are identified as vulnerable because they lack the cognitive capacity to provide informed consent, which many consider an essential requirement for participation in research. The lack of clinical trial data for children, however, makes them "therapeutic orphans" and means that pediatric prescribing decisions have been based on the extrapolation

The Science and Ethics of Antipsychotic Use in Children. http://dx.doi.org/10.1016/B978-0-12-800016-8.00005-2

of adult evidence on a case-by-case basis (Avard, Black, Samuel, Griener, & Knoppers, 2012; Shirkey, 1999; Spetie & Arnold, 2007).

Internationally, there has been an ethical zeitgeist change. No longer is the focus on protecting children from research. Today, the focus is on increasing the inclusion of children and adolescents in clinical research. It is now a requirement of many health agencies that children be included in clinical trials for medications to receive approval. The ethical impetus to include children in research is largely based on the principle of justice and concern for welfare (Avard et al., 2012; Canadian Institutes of Health Research, Natural Sciences and Engineering Research Council of Canada, & Social Sciences and Humanities Research Council of Canada, 2010). Justice pertains to the risk and benefit in research, so that the burden of research is not unfairly placed on a particular group or population, and concurrently that certain groups are not unfairly excluded from studies. In this way, the benefits and burdens of research are distributed evenly. Additionally, there is concern for welfare because children may be harmed if the only available treatments are not studied with them in mind. These concerns have prompted policy and incentives to increase pediatric clinical trials, which we review below. Moreover, there has been a push to require that clinical trial information and outcomes be made available to the public through registry databases (ICMJE Editorial, 2004). The aim of registries is to increase research transparency and access to information about clinical trials.

Currently, there is little evidence that these policies have been successful in increasing the evidence base in a way that enhances child welfare and health outcomes (Caldwell, Murphy, Butow, & Craig, 2004; Jong, van der Anker, & Choonara, 2001; Murthy et al., 2013). The aim of this chapter is to review clinical trial activity for AP research involving children (< 12 years old) and adolescents (12-18 years of age) to determine if calls for more robust research in this area have been heeded. To review the current landscape of trials, we examined trial information made available on worldwide clinical trial registries. Our findings reveal that AP clinical trial activity has steadily declined since 2010 and includes a wide variety of interventions, indications, age ranges, and outcome measures. Moreover, results from trials are often not reported in the registries, which undermine the benefits of research. We discuss the ethical implications of our findings and end with some practical suggestions for the road ahead.

Patient Safety, Ethics, and Clinical Trial Regulation

One of the first legal requirements in North America for safe medications arose as a result of the "Elixir Sulfanilamide incident." In 1937, over 100 people died after taking a liquefied version of a common antibiotic which was sweetened with diethylene glycol. This toxin was identified as poisonous after it had been released and prescribed by doctors across the country. Many of those who died were children. This tragedy provided a catalyst for the FDA Cosmetic Act of 1938, which required truthful labeling and toxicity studies of all medicines (Ballentine, 1981). It was not until the 1960s, however, that the requirement for clinical trials emerged following another tragedy: the thalidomide catastrophe. At this time, pregnant women across Europe and other parts of the world, including Canada, had been prescribed thalidomide for morning sickness. Regrettably, it later transpired that this medication caused deformities in newborn infants. The USA, however, was not affected, as a new member of the FDA team, Frances Oldham Kelsey, did not approve the drug for use in pregnant women due to a lack of substantial evidence for safety. This foresight is credited with saving American children from the negative side effects of thalidomide and inspired new legislation—the Harris-Kefauver Amendment of 1962. This amendment made the provision of safety and efficacy information mandatory for all medications and defined the distinct phases of clinical trial research (FDA News & Events, 2012).

The Push for Pediatric Clinical Trials

The United States is also a world leader in the push to encourage pediatric clinical trials. In 1997, the U.S. FDA Modernization Act incentivized pediatric research by creating a 6-month patent extension for pharmaceutical companies that carried out pediatric tests. Extending the marketing exclusivity of a drug represents a significant financial incentive for pharmaceutical companies. In the following year, further legislation was passed, mandating pediatric testing for all new drug development (Pediatric Final Rule, 1998). While this requirement was overturned in 2002, it was reinstated in 2003 under the Pediatric Research Equity Act (PREA). The requirements included in PREA were also complimented by the Best Pharmaceuticals for Children Act (BPCA: US FDA, 2002), which implemented three key activities in support of pediatric clinical trials: (1) identifying and prioritizing drugs needing study; (2) developing study requests in collaboration with health agencies; and (3) conducting studies on priority drugs if manufacturers declined to do so. Both PREA and BPCA were permanently reauthorized in 2012, with an additional consideration for research with neonates (Food and Drug Administration Reform Act of 2012). Under these new rules, the FDA has the power to impose financial penalties on pharmaceutical companies that are not forthcoming with pediatric data and has the authority to "misbrand" a drug, taking it off the market. This latter strategy, while formidable, is not considered an ideal consequence, as it would result in the denial of a drug from adult patients for whom the drug may have evidence of efficacy (Thaul, 2012).

Internationally, the World Health Assembly has also called for more research in pediatric medicine (WHO: Better Medicines for Children, 2007). In Europe, incentives of market exclusivity similar to those in the USA have also been enacted (European Medicines Agency, 2007). In contrast to the significant activities of its American and European counterparts, Canada has made little progress with regard to incentivizing pediatric clinical trials. In 2003, Health

Canada adopted International Conference on Harmonisation (ICH) guidance on pediatric clinical trials, which called for more pediatric trials to inform prescribing practices. However, this policy has no legal or incentivizing power. The recent introduction of the Canadian Clinical Trials Coordinating Centre (CCTCC) in April 2014, however, suggests a positive move toward more clinical trial requirements.

The Push for Clinical Trial Registration

Preregistration of clinical trials on publically available websites has been identified as a means to promote knowledge sharing and provide some independent oversight to the field of clinical trial research. With the goal of fostering international transparency, accountability, and the scientific rigor of clinical trials, the International Committee of Medical Journal Editors (ICJME) announced in 2004 that trial registration would be required for publication of clinical trial results in medical journals. This announcement was soon followed by the WHO International Clinical Trials Registry Platform policy in 2006, stating that trial registration is a "scientific, ethical and moral responsibility" and is required to reduce the likelihood that negative or harmful findings are hidden from public scrutiny (ARVO Editorial, 2006). Clinical trial registration on a publically available website has been a requirement for Canadian Institutes of Health Research (CIHR) funding since 2004. It has been a requirement for FDA funding since 2007 in the USA and a legal requirement for funding in the EU since 2011. The most widely used registry in the world is based in the USA: ClinicalTrials. gov. Other countries that have registries include the EU-funded clinicaltrialregister.eu, and the UK-based (but internationally focused) controlled-trials.com. Fourteen additional trial registries are listed on the WHO International Clinical Trials Registry Platform (see Appendix A for a link to this resource). To date, Canada does not have a clinical trial registry of its own. However, Health Canada does provide public access to a clinical trials database that lists all trials authorized by the agency since April 1, 2013. Since this resource is not a registry, however, it does not contain comprehensive information about each clinical trial.

Reporting of Results

In September 2008, the U.S. FDA further introduced a requirement for investigators to report trial results on ClinicalTrials.gov. In September 2009, a further requirement to report adverse effects was implemented (Section 801 of the Food and Drug Administration Amendments Act, FDAAA). FDA-applicable clinical trials now have 12 months to report their results following trial completion (ClinicalTrials.gov, accessed April 6, 2014). This requirement, however, only applies to U.S. trials initiated since September 2007. Ethical policy guidance in Canada and abroad has been updated recently to reflect this growing trend; the Tri-Council Policy Statement (Canadian Institutes of Health Research, Natural

Sciences and Engineering Research Council of Canada, & Social Sciences and Humanities Research Council of Canada, 2010) and the World Medical Association (WMA) Declaration of Helsinki (2013) now state that trial registration before recruitment is mandatory. The widespread and international acceptance of clinical trial registration that has resulted from these international initiatives provides a model of how the culture of scientific reporting can be enhanced.

MAPPING THE LANDSCAPE: CLINICAL TRIALS FOR ANTIPSYCHOTICS IN CHILDREN AND YOUTH

With these historical, legal, and ethical considerations in mind, we now review the current landscape of AP clinical trial activity in children and adolescents to identify the types and magnitude of research being conducted and the extent of results reporting on trial registries.

Methods

We accessed a total of 16 clinical trial registry databases to examine the number and types of trials for APs over time. Here, we searched for any trials involving the administration of AP medications to participants aged 18 and younger. Data from the registries were combined and screened to ensure that duplicate trials were removed and that only trials including children or adolescents and antipsychotic were examined. After excluding duplicates, 243 unique studies were identified on just three registries ClinicalTrials.gov based in the United States, clinicaltrialsregister.eu based in Europe, and controlled-trials.com, an international register based in the United Kingdom. Combined, these three registries contain information on over 199,000 clinical trials.

Information on specific age ranges was then collected for these 243 trials. This analysis resulted in the exclusion of an additional 23 trials because they did not report a lower age range or were for the study of advanced age-related conditions such as dementia or Parkinson's disease, making it difficult to ascertain if children and youth were actually included in the trial. In addition, 73 studies included participants aged over 18 years old. Here, there was concern that these trials may have been piggybacking children into a predominantly adult trial, in which child-specific factors were not reported or inadequate numbers of children were recruited to inform evidence on the safety or efficacy of APs for children (Caldwell, Murphy, Butow, & Craig, 2004). For this reason, these 73 trials were excluded from the final analysis. As of January 9, 2014, our end sample included 147 clinical trials.

For each of the 147 unique trials, we recorded the following information about the trial characteristics as reported in the registries

- Trial location
- Start date

- End date
- Trial status
- Trial sponsor/investigator
- Trial design
- Trial phase*
- Sample size
- Age ranges of participants
- Health conditions under study
- Antipsychotics under study
- Outcome measures used
- Adverse event measures
- Presence of reported results

Results

Our findings are summarized in Tables 5.1 and 5.2. Table 5.1 displays key trial characteristics according to status (active, discontinued, and complete). In Table 5.2, key trial characteristics are displayed as a function of study sponsor (pharmaceutical industry, academic/health institutions, or a collaboration of both).

Trial location: The majority of trials (78%, $n = 115$) were based in the USA, and the rest were located in Europe (11%, $n = 16$), Asia (5%, $n = 7$), Canada (3%, $n = 5$), and Central and South America (2%, $n = 3$).

Trial start/end dates: The earliest registered trial dated back to 1993 and the number of clinical trials being initiated with children rose steadily until peaking in 2004 when trial registration was introduced as a requirement for publication (ICMJE Editorial, 2004). Since the FDA mandated trial registration in 2007, the number of trials has fluctuated, with another peak occurring in 2010 (see Figure 5.1). The completion date for trials (actual for completed trials, expected for trials that are not yet complete) followed a similar pattern, with

---

* Note: In the Harris-Kefauver Amendment (1962), four trial phases were identified: Phase 1 trials study drug safety in humans, and involve few participants because risks are uncertain and therapeutic benefit is not intended. Phase 2 trials study the dosage levels required for an effect. If a drug has passed phases 1 and 2, it may then be tested in a phase 3 trial, which studies the safety and efficacy of a drug against the best available treatment or a placebo. If a drug is shown to be sufficiently safe and effective in phase 3 trials, it may be approved. Once approved and made available on the market, ongoing drug safety and efficacy monitoring is carried out through phase 4 trials. A relatively new category of trials known as phase 2/3 trials has also been introduced. These trials combine the dosage element of phase 2 and the safety and efficacy goals of phase 3 trials. These types of trials are increasingly accepted as more efficient and are deemed to be as robust as carrying out two distinct trials. In this way, phase 2/3 trials are considered ethically sound as they reduce the burden of clinical trials by requiring fewer participants to enroll (Thall, 2008). In most instances, children are not included in phase 1 or phase 2 clinical trials, as there is a higher level of risk with minimal expected benefit. Phase 3 trials are, however, required for pediatric approval, and phase 4 research is encouraged to identify any adverse effects after the drug has reached the market.

TABLE 5.1 Key Characteristics of Active, Discontinued, and Completed Clinical Trials for APs in Children and Youth Between 1993 and 2013

	Total	Active		Discontinued		Completed	
	n = 147	n = 36	(25%)	n = 11	(7%)	n = 100	(68%)
Registry							
ClinicalTrials.gov	139	32	23%	10	7%	97	70%
Clinicaltrialsregister.eu	6	4	67%	1	17%	1	17%
ISRCTN	2	–	–	–	–	2	100%
Location							
USA	115	18	16%	10	9%	87	76%
EU	16	9	56%	1	6%	6	38%
Asia	7	5	71%	–	–	2	29%
Canada	5	2	40%	–	–	3	60%
Central & South America	3	1	33%	–	–	2	67%
Africa	1	1	100%	–	–	–	–
Sponsor							
Academic/health institutions	58	21	36%	3	5%	34	59%
Pharmaceutical industry	67	14	21%	5	7%	48	72%
Collaboration (both)	22	1	5%	3	14%	18	82%

Continued

TABLE 5.1 Key Characteristics of Active, Discontinued, and Completed Clinical Trials for APs in Children and Youth Between 1993 and 2013—Cont'd

	Total	Active		Discontinued		Completed	
	n = 147	n = 36	(25%)	n = 11	(7%)	n = 100	(68%)
Design							
RCT	71	21	30%	5	7%	45	63%
Open label	64	13	20%	5	8%	46	72%
Observational	5	1	20%	1	20%	3	60%
Placebo included in trial	38	9	24%	4	11%	25	66%
Behavioral intervention	5	2	40%	–	–	3	60%
Trial phase							
Phase 1	4	1	25%	0	0%	3	75%
Phase 2	16	2	13%	1	6%	13	81%
Phase 2/3	4	2	50%	1	25%	1	25%
Phase 3	65	15	23%	4	6%	46	71%
Phase 4	32	6	19%	3	9%	23	72%
Not specified	26	10	38%	2	8%	14	54%
Sample size							
Small (1-99)	77	16	21%	5	6%	56	73%
Medium (100-299)	43	9	21%	3	7%	31	72%

	Total	Active		Discontinued		Completed	
	n=147	n=36	(25%)	n=11	(7%)	n=100	(68%)
Large (300-999)	15	5	33%	0	0%	10	67%
Not specified	11	6	55%	3	27%	2	18%
Age							
Childhood (age 2-11)	10	1	10%	0	0%	9	90%
Adolescents (age 12-18)	39	10	26%	3	8%	26	7%
All (age 2-18)	98	25	26%	8	8%	65	66%
Conditions							
ADHD	7	2	29%	1	14%	4	57%
ASD	26	8	31%	–	–	18	69%
Bipolar	32	3	9%	5	16%	24	75%
Conduct	8	1	13%	–	–	7	87%
Eating disorder	3	2	67%	–	–	1	33%
Mood disorder	2	1	50%	–	–	1	50%
Multiple conditions	28	4	14%	1	4%	23	82%
Psychosis	2	2	100%	–	–	–	–
Schizophrenia	19	3	16%	2	10%	14	74%
Tourette's/tic disorder	10	4	40%	2	20%	5	50%
Other—not psychiatric	9	5	56%	1	11%	3	33%

Continued

TABLE 5.1 Key Characteristics of Active, Discontinued, and Completed Clinical Trials for APs in Children and Youth Between 1993 and 2013—Cont'd

	Total	Active		Discontinued		Completed	
	n = 147	n = 36	(25%)	n = 11	(7%)	n = 100	(68%)
Antipsychotics							
Aripiprazole	42	13	31%	3	7%	26	62%
Asenpine	5	1	20%	–	–	4	80%
Clozapine	1	–	–	–	–	1	100%
Iloperidone	1	1	100%	–	–	–	–
Olanzapine	10	3	30%	–	–	7	70%
Paliperidone	6	1	17%	1	17%	4	67%
Quetiapine	10	2	20%	–	–	8	80%
Risperidone	28	6	21%	–	–	22	79%
Ziprasidone	13	–	–	4	31%	9	69%
Multiple APs	16	4	25%	1	6%	11	69%
Typical APs	8	3	38%	–	–	5	63%
Not specified	2	1	50%	1	50%	–	–
Reported results on ct.gov							
Has results	30	–	–	4	13%	26	87%
No results	115	36	31%	7	6%	72	63%

TABLE 5.2 Key Characteristics of Pharmaceutical, Academic, and Collaborative Clinical Trials for APs in Children and Youth Between 1993 and 2013

	Total		Pharmaceutical		Collaboration		Academic/Health	
	n = 147		n = 67	(46%)	n = 22	(15%)	n = 58	(39%)
Registry								
ClinicalTrials.gov	139		63	45%	22	16%	54	39%
Clinicaltrialsregister.eu	6		4	67%	–	–	2	33%
ISRCTN	2		–	–	–	–	2	100%
Location								
USA	115		53	46%	21	18%	41	36%
EU	16		7	44%	1	6%	8	50%
Asia	7		6	86%	–	–	1	14%
Canada	5		1	20%	–	–	4	80%
Central & South America	3		–	–	–	–	3	100%
Africa	1		–	–	–	–	1	100%
Status								
Active	36		14	39%	1	3%	21	58%
Complete	100		48	48%	18	18%	34	34%

Continued

TABLE 5.2 Key Characteristics of Pharmaceutical, Academic, and Collaborative Clinical Trials for APs in Children and Youth Between 1993 and 2013—Cont'd

	Total	Pharmaceutical		Collaboration		Academic/Health	
	n=147	n=67	(46%)	n=22	(15%)	n=58	(39%)
Discontinued	11	5	45%	3	27%	3	27%
Design							
RCT	71	37	52%	6	8%	28	39%
Open label	64	29	45%	14	22%	21	33%
Observational	5	1	20%	1	20%	3	60%
Placebo included in trial	38	21	55%	3	8%	14	37%
Behavioral intervention	5	1	20%	–	–	4	80%
Phase							
Phase 1	4	3	75%	0	0%	1	25%
Phase 2	16	4	25%	5	31%	7	44%
Phase 2/3	4	1	25%	2	50%	1	25%
Phase 3	65	48	74%	7	11%	10	15%
Phase 4	32	7	22%	5	16%	20	63%

	Total	Pharmaceutical		Collaboration		Academic/Health	
	n=147	n=67	(46%)	n=22	(15%)	n=58	(39%)
Not specified	26	4	15%	3	12%	19	73%
Sample size							
Small (1-99)	77	16	21%	21	27%	40	52%
Medium (100-299)	43	33	77%	–	–	10	23%
Large (300-999)	15	10	67%	–	–	5	33%
Missing sample size	11	8	73%	1	9%	2	18%
Age							
Childhood (age 2-11)	10	0	0%	1	10%	9	90%
Adolescents (age 12-18)	39	23	59%	5	13%	10	26%
All (age 2-18)	98	44	45%	16	16%	38	39%
Conditions							
ADHD	6	1	17%	2	33%	3	50%
ASD	26	9	35%	5	19%	12	46%
Bipolar	32	12	38%	7	22%	13	41%
Conduct	8	4	50%	2	25%	2	25%
Eating disorder	3	–	–	–	–	3	100%

Continued

TABLE 5.2 Key Characteristics of Pharmaceutical, Academic, and Collaborative Clinical Trials for APs in Children and Youth Between 1993 and 2013—cont'd

	Total	Pharmaceutical		Collaboration		Academic/Health	
	n = 147	n = 67	(46%)	n = 22	(15%)	n = 58	(39%)
Mood disorder	2	–		1	50%	1	50%
Multiple conditions	25	16	64%	2	8%	7	28%
Psychosis,	2	–		–		2	100%
Schizophrenia	19	17	89%	–		2	11%
Tourette's/tic disorder	10	6	60%	1	10%	3	30%
Other—not psychiatric	8	–		1	13%	7	88%
Antipsychotic							
Aripiprazole	42	22	52%	12	29%	8	19%
Asenpine	5	5	100%	–		–	
Clozapine	1	–		–		1	100%
Iloperidone	1	1	100%	–		–	
Olanzapine	10	5	50%	–		5	50%
Paliperidone	6	5	83%	–		1	17%

	Total	Pharmaceutical		Collaboration		Academic/Health	
	n = 147	n = 67	(46%)	n = 22	(15%)	n = 58	(39%)
Quetiapine	10	4	40%	2	20%	4	40%
Risperidone	28	13	46%	1	4%	14	50%
Ziprasidone	13	7	54%	4	31%	2	15%
Multiple APs	16	2	13%	2	13%	12	75%
Typical APs	8	2	25%	–	–	6	75%
Not specified	2	–	–	–	–	2	100%
Reported results on Clinicaltrials.gov							
Has results	30	21	70%	2	7%	7	23%
No results	115	46	40%	20	17%	49	43%

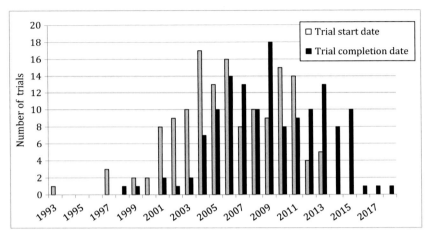

FIGURE 5.1   Numbers of trials started and ended over time.

the highest number of trials ending in 2009. Overall, trials took anywhere from 0 to 133 months to complete, with an average of 38 months (just over 3 years) between trial start and end dates.

Trial status: A quarter of the trials (25%, $n=36$) were active as of January 2014, while 68% ($n=100$) were complete and 7% ($n=11$) were discontinued. This discontinued category includes trials that were terminated ($n=6$), withdrawn ($n=3$), prematurely ended ($n=1$), or suspended ($n=1$). See Table 5.1 for further details.

Trial sponsor/investigator: Information about the type of sponsor for each trial was categorized by three variables: academic/health institution, pharmaceutical industry, or jointly sponsored by both (collaboration). Pharmaceutical companies were listed as the sponsor for 46% of trials ($n=67$), closely followed by academic/health institutions (39%, $n=58$ trials), and the remaining were sponsored by a collaboration of both (15%, $n=22$ trials). While collaborations accounted for 15% of all trials, they accounted for 27% of all discontinued trials. In contrast, academic/health institutions accounted for 39% of all trials, but 58% of active trials as of January 2014.

It is notable that almost one-third of industry-sponsored trials (31%) involved only two pharmaceutical companies: Johnson & Johnson group (16%, $n=23$) and Otsuka (15%, $n=22$). Bristol Meyer's Squib was the third most active pharmaceutical company, involved in 10% ($n=15$) of all trials; however the majority of these ($n=13$) were collaborative studies with an academic/health institution (see Figure 5.2).

Trial design: Almost all (97%, $n=142$) trials were interventional, with 3% ($n=5$) listed as observational. Nearly half (48%, $n=71$) of the interventional trials were randomized controlled trials RCTs, with double blinding, whereas 44% ($n=64$) of trials were open-label, most of which were not randomized ($n=50$). Approximately one-quarter of trials (26%, $n=38$) included a placebo control group, and 3% ($n=5$) listed a behavioral intervention as part of the trial design.

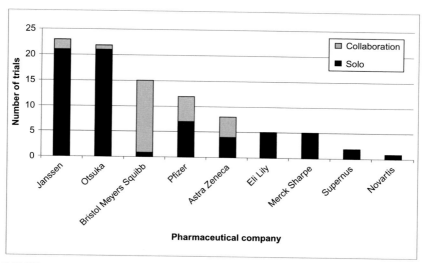

FIGURE 5.2   Janssen and Otsuka pharmaceutical companies are leaders in AP research involving children and youth.

Trial phase: Phase information was missing for 14% ($n=21$) of registered trials. Of those trials that reported phase, almost half were described as phase 3 (44%, $n=65$), followed by phase 4 (22%, $n=32$), and phase 2 (11%, $n=16$). There were minimal phase 2/3 and phase 1 trials. Table 5.1 and 5.3 provide further details on trial phase.

Sample size: Over one-half (52%, $n=77$) of the trials were small (under 100 participants), 29% ($n=43$) were medium sized (100-299) and 10% ($n=15$) were large (> 300). Information on sample size was missing for 7% of trials ($n=11$; of which two were indicated as complete). Information on sample size was available for four of the five observational trials, all of which were small (see Table 5.3 for details). Overall, medium-size phase 3 trials were the most common type of trial registered (20% of all trials; $n=29$).

Age ranges of participants: The age range of participants across all trials was from 2 to 18 years, with age ranges spanning an average of 8 years (for example an age range of 2-10 or 10-18 years). Since there are vast developmental differences between very young children and older youth, we categorized trials according to age groups: childhood (ages 2-11 years), adolescent (ages 12-18 years), and trials that included both children and adolescents (ages 2-18 years). One trial involved only early childhood participants, 2% involved middle childhood, and 26% involved adolescents only (age 12 and up). Most trials involved more than one age category, with one-third of the trials including children from all age categories.

Health conditions under study: Of the 147 trials, the most common condition under study was bipolar disorder (22%, $n=32$), followed by autism spectrum disorder (ASD) (18%; $n=26$) and schizophrenia (13%; $n=19$). Eighteen percent

TABLE 5.3 Medium Sized, Phase 3 Trials Were the Most Common

	Total by Phase	Small Sample (0-99)	Medium Sample (100-299)	Large Sample (300-999)	Missing n
Phase 1	4	3	1	–	–
Phase 2	16	13	2	–	1
Phase 2/3	4	3	–	–	1
Phase 3	65	22	29	11	3
Phase 4	32	20	8	3	1
Missing	21	13	3	1	4
Observational	5	4	–	–	1
Total by size	147	78	43	15	11

($n=25$) of the studies involved multiple disorders, with more than half of these (52%, $n=13$) studying "bipolar and psychosis." See Table 5.1 for the full list of conditions that were studied.

Antipsychotics under study: The most common antipsychotic drugs under study were: aripiprazole (28%, $n=41$), risperidone (21%, $n=31$), and ziprasidone (9%, $n=13$). Eleven percent of the trials ($n=16$) involved multiple treatment arms comparing different APs. Only 5% ($n=8$) of the interventional trials involved typical APs. See Table 5.1 for full list.

Intervention combinations: Table 5.4 contains information about the most frequent conditions and APs under study for identification of common intervention combinations. As displayed, there is little consistency. The most frequent combination was the use of aripiprazole for the treatment of ASD (9%, $n=13$), followed by risperidone for ASD (6%, $n=9$) and aripiprazole for Tourette's/tic disorders (6%, $n=8$). Tourette's/tic disorders had little variation in APs, in that aripiprazole was tested in 80% of the trials. In contrast, 10 different APs were studied for bipolar disorder and 8 APs were used in schizophrenia research.

Outcome measures: The outcome measures used in the 147 clinical trials were primarily clinician-rated standardized measures. The most widely used tool was the Clinical Global Impressions (CGIs) scale, used in 41% of trials ($n=61$). The CGIs scale was specifically developed by the National Institute of Mental Health to be administered by non-researcher clinicians to quantify and track patient progress. It includes clinician-rated measures of the presence, frequency, and impact of clinical symptoms. Two types of CGI score were reported in our sample; CGI-Improvement and CGI-Severity. Additionally, two adapted CGI scales were used as outcome measures, with eight studies using the CGI-Bipolar and five using CGI-Tourette's Syndrome scales (see Table 5.5). The Youth Mania Rating Scale (YMRS) was used in 20% of trials ($n=29$), mostly in studies of bipolar disorder, and the Aberrant Behavior Checklist (ABC) was used in 14% ($n=21$) of all trials. The CGI measure was most frequently used in ASD studies (69%, $n=18$), and next was the ABC tool (65%, $n=17$). The Positive and Negative Syndrome Scale (PANNS) (63%, $n=12$) and CGI (53%, $n=10$) were typically used for measuring schizophrenia-related outcomes.

Adverse event measures: Forty-seven percent of trials ($n=69$) reported using measures to monitor adverse physical effects, including physical markers (such as Body Mass Index and blood pressure). Some also included standardized measures, such as the Abnormal Involuntary Movement Scale, Barnes-Akathisia Rating Scale, and Simpson-Angus Scale.

Reporting of results in clinical trial registries: Out of 147 trials, 100 were reported as complete and 11 as discontinued by January 2014. Only 27% ($n=30$) of the 111 trials that had ended posted results on ClinicalTrials.gov. Since the reporting of results was not mandatory for trials prior to 2007, we examined reporting rates before and after 2007 (trials ending after December of 2012 were not included as they were still within the 12-month reporting moratorium at time of our analysis in January 2014). A total of 16 applicable trials were identified,

TABLE 5.4 Frequency of Trials for Common Intervention Combinations in AP Clinical Trials for Children and Youth

	Arip	Risp	Zipr	Olan	Quet	Total	#APs Tested/Condition[a]
ASD	13	9	1	2	–	26	5
Bipolar disorder	6	3	6	2	6	32	10
Tourette's/tic disorders	8	–	–	–	–	10	2
Schizophrenia	5	2	3	1	1	19	8
Conduct issues	1	6	1	–	–	8	3
ADHD	2	4	–	–	1	7	3
Total	41	31	13	10	10		
Number of conditions[b]	8	8	4	5	5		

Abbreviations: Arip, aripiprazole; Risp, risperidone; Zipr, ziprasidone; Olan, olanzapine; Quet, quetiapine.
[a]Values reflect all APs tested across clinical trials, including APs not listed in table.
[b]Values reflect numbers of all conditions studied across clinical trials, including conditions not listed in table.

TABLE 5.5 Type and Frequency of Outcome Measures Reported as a Function of Mental Health Condition in AP Clinical Trials for Children and Youth

Condition	Outcome Measures							
	YMRS	CGI	ABC	PANNS	CGAS	CDRS	Incl. ADRs	Other (n)
Bipolar disorder	23	9	–	–	4	9	11	CGI-BP (8)
ASD	–	18	17	–	1	–	10	–
Schizophrenia	–	10	–	12	6	3	9	–
Conduct issues	–	6	2	–	1	–	4	–
ADHD	–	4	–	1	2	–	3	ADHD-RS (3)
Tourette's/tic disorders	–	3	–	–	–	1	3	CGI-TS (5) YGTSS (8)
Multiple & other	8	11	2	5	5	2	69	–
Total	29	61	21	18	19	15	61	

Abbreviations: ABC, Aberrant Behavior Checklist; ADHD-RS, ADHD Rating Scale; CDRS, Children's Depression Rating Scale; CGAS, Children's Global Assessment Scale; CGI, Clinical Global Impressions Scale (including Severity and Improvement); CGI-BP, Clinical Global Impressions Scale-BiPolar; CGI-TS, Clinical Global Impressions Scale-Tourette's Syndrome; Incl. ADRs, Inclusion of measurements (not specified here) for adverse reactions; PANNS, Positive and Negative Syndrome Scale; YGTSS, Yale Global Tic Severity Scale; YMRS, Youth Mania Rating Scale.

with only 6 reporting results in the registry by January 2014. Surprisingly, the majority of trials that reported results (63%; $n = 19$) were initiated prior to the 2007 requirement date. Most studies that had reported results were conducted by the pharmaceutical industry (70%, $n = 21$), while just two were collaborative investigations (7%) and seven (23%) were by academic/health institutions.

REFLECTIONS ON THE CURRENT STATE OF PEDIATRIC CLINICAL TRIALS FOR ANTIPSYCHOTICS

Given the complexities involved with pediatric clinical trials and the use of antipsychotic drugs for children, the finding of 147 registered trials is perhaps higher than expected. However, the results presented describe a varied landscape of registered trials for a wide range of antipsychotic drugs and psychiatric conditions that make interpretations about the efficacy of APs for any one condition difficult. Moreover, there has been a steady drop off in the number of new trials since 2009. These findings indicate that while some progress is being made, more research needs to be done to inform the treatment decisions of patients, families, and their doctors. Below, we identify key ethical considerations for our most salient findings.

The Landscape of Clinical Trial Activity

Our data indicate that the USA is the location of most clinical trial activity for APs in children and youth, with sponsorship by the pharmaceutical industry leading the way. Financial incentives in the USA (1998) and in the European Union (2007) for the pharmaceutical industry to conduct research in pediatric populations may account for the increase in the number of trials registered between 2002 and 2009, however it is unclear why activity has dropped off since then. Potential influences on clinical trial initiation may include, among other factors, government policy, ethics board requirements, market saturation, success of another drug, prevalence of a condition, clinical burden of a condition, patent expiration of a drug, sales in adult populations, or new evidence about the condition or drug.

Others have shown that the pharmaceutical industry enrolls more people in its trials and funds more trials on antipsychotics (Bourgeois, Murthy, & Mandl, 2010) than academia—a finding that is supported by the results reported here. Pharmaceutical companies carried out three times as many medium-size trials (100-299 participants), and twice as many with large sample sizes (>300) as academic/health institutions. The pattern of who is taking the lead in pediatric clinical trials may be changing, however, given that academic/health institutions are responsible for almost 60% of active trials as of January 2014. This may be a reflection of withdrawal of the pharmaceutical companies in response to the approval of some APs. It may also more generally reflect the unexpected and widespread pullout from neuroscience research by the pharmaceutical industry (Amara, Grillner, Insel, Nutt, & Tsumoto, 2011). For pharmaceutical companies, there are also financial implications of making proprietary knowledge available to competitors on registries, especially in the early stages of research (phases 1 and 2 trials). Some have warned that the competitive advantage that ultimately drives drug sales may be eliminated if safeguards are not put in place to protect intellectual property (Campbell Alliance, 2005). A chief concern is that incentives for companies to develop new drugs will be reduced. One proposed solution is to only require companies to provide the public with a general overview of the trial protocol. In this case, detailed information would be filed but kept confidential until the study was completed (Campbell Alliance, 2005).

Despite lagging industry involvement in recent years, pharmaceutical sponsors were responsible for 39% of all pediatric clinical trials on APs found in the registries. This highlights the significant role of large pharmaceutical companies in clinical trials. Bristol Meyer's Squibb was primarily involved in collaborative investigations, and partners with the Japanese-based company Otsuka. They jointly market and sell aripiprazole, as an example. While it is beyond the scope of this chapter to identify reasons for collaboration, it is likely that resources, geographical location, and business models are involved. It is clear, however, that there is little variety among the main actors in this field, and thus a less competitive marketplace.

Finally, the success of APs in treating schizophrenia and bipolar disorders in youth may have heightened motivation to establish their effectiveness for treatment of other conditions. The diversity of indications and AP treatments under investigation highlights a field where researchers are examining a wide range of medications for a wide range of disorders. Aripiprazole, for example, has been tested with eight different conditions, from psychosis to behavioral disorders to tic disorders. While this approach may represent a desire to identify what works best, it creates difficulties for practitioners trying to interpret the best course of action. It is possible that many unique trial combinations were not replicated due to a negative outcome, and that the most commonly paired conditions and APs were correlated with effectiveness.

Overall, it is promising that there may be results from up to 36 currently active trials in the coming years. In our sample, completed trials took an average of 3 years from start to end date. This trial length does not represent the length of time that any participant was taking the drug, however, as drug administration is usually a matter of weeks. The 3-year timeframe likely reflects the time needed to enroll a large enough sample size of participants and provide adequate follow-up for participants.

Developmental Gaps

We found very few registered trials in early childhood, a population for which there is a growing concern. Prescription trends are on the rise for preschool children in particular, who are at a uniquely "plastic" age (Arnold, 2001; Spetie

& Arnold, 2007). Trials in our review often recruited youth from a wide range of ages, with the average age span of 8 years between participants in the same study. Few trials included only children, with most trials grouping children and adolescents together. Given the evolving developmental state of children, it is unclear whether information about young people aged 6 and 14 years is comparable or useful when combined. Immense physiological and psychological changes occur throughout childhood. Specific information about the impact of APs for children at key developmental periods, such as early childhood, middle childhood, and adolescence is necessary to guide clinicians in making treatment recommendations. It is also notable that we had to exclude 73 trials from our analysis because they included both children and adults in the study design. In some of these cases, children were listed under inclusion criteria for dementia or Parkinson's research. Ultimately, we had to exclude these trials from our analysis due to concerns about piggybacking, the practice of using a primary study to support multiple ancillary studies. Given the often non-discriminate inclusion of young children in AP studies with older adolescents or adults, it is possible that their participation may be a nod to inclusion rather than a meaningful investigation of whether or not a given drug is effective in this population. Generally, including children in adult clinical trials is not desirable, unless there are provisions for appropriate sample sizes and statistical analysis. Therefore, it is an ethical concern that the contribution of children included in those studies is undermined and that they are exposed to risk with no social benefit. According to recent guidelines published under the Standards for Research in Child Health (StaR) initiative, which seeks to enhance the quality, ethics, and reliability of pediatric research, trial designs must include meaningful age categories that are associated with the conditions under study (Williams et al., 2012).

The Strength of Evidence

Currently, double-blind RCTs are the gold standard method for identifying safety and efficacy parameters for medications and are usually required before a drug is approved for sale. In a trial in which there is more than one treatment being tested, it is best practice to randomly assign participants to a treatment group to avoid the potential for biasing the sample. Biasing could occur if researchers assign patients to different groups based on confounding characteristics, such as the severity of their illness or their response to previous treatments. Once assigned to groups, participants may (for open-label trials) or may not be made aware of which treatment they are receiving. Not telling participants which group they are in is called blinding, and it is a process invoked to reduce the potential for a placebo effect. Given that patient expectation of treatment can lead to positive outcomes, placebo groups are often included so that researchers can determine if the active drug under investigation produced true effects. Although limited, there is some evidence that children are more likely to display a stronger placebo effect than adults (Weimer, et al., 2013). To further reduce the confound potential, some trial designs include a further element of blinding in which the researchers involved are also unaware of which treatment the participant is receiving (a double-blind design). Double-blind, randomized, placebo-controlled trials are the most valid and robust form of clinical trial at present to assess drug efficacy and safety. However, researchers must keep in mind that randomly assigning participants to a treatment or placebo control group is only ethically acceptable when there is clinical equipoise—a situation where all treatments being offered in the study are considered equal because there is no certainty that any one treatment is better or worse than the others, including the placebo (Freedman, 1987; Sugarman, 2002). Simply put, it would be harmful, and therefore unethical, to deny a patient access to a known beneficial treatment.

In our analysis, double-blind RCT designs were used in one-half of the registered trials. Of these, half included a placebo arm. Overall, this is encouraging, given that drug approvals from federal health agencies necessitate robust levels of evidence. The finding that placebo groups were used for only one-quarter of the trials suggests that clinical equipoise considerations may be common in AP studies. Also common was the use of non-randomized open-label designs. Open-label trials may be appropriate for comparing two very similar treatments to determine which is most effective. The high prevalence of non-randomized open-label trials suggests that patients, families, and doctors are deciding which treatment a child is going to receive, likely to minimize the potential for harm. Treatment preferences and group assignment may be based on previous experience with a specific treatment, either positive or negative. Although this kind of trial design introduces a certain degree of bias, it may be more appropriate to ensure that participants comply with treatment.

Sample size is also an important indicator of the strength of findings. Although there is no consensus on the ideal sample size for different trial phases, phase 3 trials often recruit over 100 participants and can include potentially thousands of people (Evans & Ildstad, 2001; Friedman, Furberg & DeMets, 1996; Piantadosi, 1997; Schuster & Powers, 2005). Here, clinical trial activity mainly revolved around phase 3 (safety and efficacy) trials, with almost half of trials recruiting fewer than 100 children and adolescents. This is not surprising given that pediatric clinical trials tend to be smaller, either by design, to avoid placing an unnecessary burden on this vulnerable population, or by circumstance because of difficulties with recruitment. For instance, there is a smaller participant pool to recruit from, due to the smaller age range, as well as a lower incidence of disease among children. Small trials, however, run the risk of lacking sufficient statistical power to identify a treatment effect and detect less common adverse effects. Thus, sample size is an important consideration for ethically robust clinical trial designs.

Furthermore, we found that phases 3 and 4 trials involved a larger number of participants than phases 1 and 2 trials. This is ethically sound as it is not required to put children at risk, and information about drug safety is better gleaned from adult studies, when possible. It is concerning, however, that there was missing information on the trial phase in 14% of cases, and, more worryingly, on trial size in 7% of cases. Sharing this information in trial registries is crucial to the integrity of the clinical trial.

Uniformity in Outcome Measures

Kumar, Datta, Wright, Furtado, and Russell (2013) highlight a need for uniform reporting in future clinical trials, so that trials can be compared and contrasted. In our analysis, the CGIs scale was used frequently, which facilitates future comparisons among clinical trial results. It is also useful to the field that there was some consistency in the condition-specific measures used: YMRS for bipolar and PANNS for schizophrenia, for example. These allow for individual trial comparisons and later systematic reviews. Few studies listed biological or physical measures as outcomes, except in relation to adverse effects. Fortunately, most clinical trials from our sample did measure adverse effects. However, the finding that physician and parent reports are primarily used to assess outcomes for child psychiatric conditions reinforces the importance of double-blindness in these clinical trials, particularly when the outcome measure is a report of perceived behavioral and emotional symptoms in a child.

Gaps in Results Reporting

To reap the full benefits of research, data from clinical trials need to be shared and translated to the general public. This latter requirement is being increasingly recognized as an essential aspect of the clinical trial process. However, the reporting of trial outcomes is often incomplete (Chan, Krleza-Ieric, Schmid, & Altman, 2004). Studies report publication rates of findings from clinical trials to be between 50% and 70% (Jones et al., 2013; Lee, Bacchetti, & Sim, 2008; Ross, Mulvey, Hines, Nissen, & Krumholz, 2009), with higher publication rates for larger trials and trials with positive results (Hopewell, Loudon, Clarke, Oxman, & Dickersin, 2009; Lee et al., 2008; Song et al., 2010). For trials that do get published, the process can take up to 2 years (Ross et al., 2009). Up to one-quarter of trials do not publish their results anywhere (Jones et al., 2013), a result reflected in this study.

Gaps in reporting are concerning given recent evidence suggesting that unpublished clinical trial data would change the efficacy outcomes of FDA-approved drugs (Hart, Lundh, & Bero, 2012). One reason for the lack of reporting is that scientists are more inclined to publish studies about interventions that have positive results, and, indeed, positive results are more likely to be accepted for publication in a peer-reviewed journal (Hopewell et al., 2009). The consequences of publication bias can have tangible impacts on patient care and the distribution of healthcare resources. Time and money may be wasted on inappropriate treatments and preclude patients from receiving more effective treatments in a timely manner. The importance of communication of negative results is validated by two core ethical principles that underpin policies for the ethical conduct of research involving humans, respect for persons and concern for welfare. The principle of respect requires that adequate efforts be made to ensure that the contributions of research participants result in generalizable knowledge. For example, some people may choose to take part in a clinical trial for the benefit of others with the same disorder; non-publication of results undermines this. Concern for welfare requires that research evidence be shared to spare patients from ineffective treatments and to prevent the squandering of finite resources on similar research (WMA: Declaration of Helsinki, Revision V, 1996; Canadian Institutes of Health Research, Natural Sciences and Engineering Research Council of Canada, & Social Sciences and Humanities Research Council of Canada, 2010).

Less than one-third of the studies in our sample reported their results in the registry. Surprisingly, those that did provide results did so prior to the FDA making it a requirement in 2008. Here, pharmaceutical industry trials were more likely to report results, which is in line with findings from previous studies showing that industry-funded trials report results more often than non-industry trials (Prayle et al., 2011). This is likely because noncompliance may result in lengthy delays of FDA approval of drugs.

One reason for failure to report findings may be that the 12-month reporting moratorium is too short, especially for academic investigators who have limited personnel and funding to carry out extensive data analysis within a 1-year timeframe. Our results suggest that academic institutions are now taking the lead in research. Since 2006, the majority of active clinical trials (60%) have been initiated by academic sponsors. Ordinarily, academic researchers aim to publish their findings in peer-reviewed journals, which can take considerable time. Peer-reviewed publications are the currency of academic research and ensure adequate interpretation of results. Publication decisions by journal editors, however, may take several months owing to lengthy peer-review processes. In some cases, extra delays may occur when researchers must resubmit their findings for additional peer review following initial rejection. To further enable the reporting of results in trial registries, the FDA should consider extending the reporting deadline. It should be noted, however, that the FDAAA rule allows for reporting delays and deadline extensions under certain conditions (visit http://clinicaltrials.gov/ct2/manage-recs/fdaaa for a detailed list of conditions). Notably, it is clearly emphasized that "pending publication is not considered good cause for an extension." Unfortunately, we were not able to determine if absent reporting in our sample was due to extension requests or noncompliance.

Today, there also remain concerns that the knowledge gained from research is not being shared internationally. Peterson et al. (2011) raised concerns that U.S.-based pharmaceutical companies are not providing pediatric safety and efficacy information to Health Canada. This omission renders some medications off-label in Canada, despite their approval in the USA. For instance, the USA has approved risperidone (2006) and aripiprazole (2009) for the treatment of ir-ritability associated with autism in children as young as 6 years old. In addition, risperidone (2007), aripiprazole (2007, 2008), olanzapine (2009), and quetiap-ine (2009) have all been approved for short-term treatment of schizophrenia in adolescents aged 13-17 years and for short-term treatment of manic or mixed episodes of bipolar I disorder in children aged 10-17 years. In contrast, Canada has only approved aripiprazole for the treatment of schizophrenia or bipolar disorder in adolescents. The difference in approval perhaps has more to do with policy and the sharing of pediatric information than a lack of clinical trial data. Indeed, risperidone, aripiprazole, olanzapine, and quetiapine were the most commonly studied drugs in registered clinical trials, which presumably led to their approval by the FDA for treating autism, psychosis, and bipolar disorder in young people once effectiveness had been established. Our findings support this assertion, given that the majority of trials involving aripiprazole and risperidone took place prior to their approval for these indications by the FDA.

Finally, a main goal of registries is to allow the public and healthcare pro-fessionals access to results so that they may become better informed about treatment options. However, results in registries are often reported without lay summaries or interpretations of the data. This can lead to misinterpretation of the findings. Ongoing reviews of reported results in registries, similar to those provided by the Cochrane Collaboration, are needed to maximize the benefits of research.

Recruitment and Willingness to Participate in Research

One of the benefits of clinical trial registration is that it allows the public ac-cess to information on active clinical trials, which may promote awareness of and participation in research (Zarin et al., 2013). At present (October 2014), ClinicalTrials.gov lists over 800 mental health studies that are actively recruit-ing participants under the age of 18 years. For patients or families wishing to find out how to participate in these studies, contact information and location sites for each trial are provided in the registry, along with the following state-ment: "Choosing to participate in a study is an important personal decision. Talk with your doctor and family members or friends about deciding to join a study. To learn more about this study, you or your doctor may contact the study research staff using the Contacts provided below. For general information, see Learn About Clinical Studies." To date, however, no research has been con-ducted to determine the impact of registries on awareness and willingness to enroll children in clinical trials. Indeed, information posted about AP trials on registries may be difficult for individuals with limited science backgrounds to interpret and may ultimately serve to confuse rather than enlighten members of the general public.

Moreover, it remains unclear if the social benefits of registries (i.e., increased transparency and the sharing of clinical trial data) are clearly understood by the general public or if this knowledge would significantly motivate families to participate in research. There is a public perception that clinical research does not involve therapeutic benefit, leading some parents and doctors to prefer routine clinical care, even if it involves off-label treatment, to enrolling a child in an experiment (Caldwell et al., 2004). Indeed, the goal of medical treatment is to improve the health of current patients, whereas medical research seeks to promote generalizable knowledge to improve the health of future patients (Beck & Azari, 1998). This discrepancy between the personal and social benefits may explain why parents are more accepting of off-label prescriptions while reluctant to enroll their child in a clinical trial where the same medication is being tested.

Informed Consent

Other ethical challenges that emerge in pediatric research include communicating effectively with parents and children about the research process and obtaining informed consent or assent (Koelch, Schnoor, & Fegert, 2008). In pediatric trials, informed consent is typically obtained from a parent or guardian (similar to the concept of "parental permission" in the U.S. context; Committee on Bioethics, 1995), along with assent from the child if appropriate. This is judged to be an acceptable compromise because parents are most often in the best position to weigh the risks and benefits of their child's enrollment in a clinical trial and are assumed to act in their child's best interest. The threshold of benefit to a child may also need to be greater for a parent to expose her or his child to a perhaps unnecessary risk (Bavdekar, 2013; Wendler, Rackoff, Emanuel, & Grady, 2002). The Belmont Report (1979) also identifies situations where the permission of both parents is required for a child to take part in research; namely, where there is some risk to the child and no direct benefit. Given the potential for adverse events related to AP use, parents and children (if possible) who participate in these studies must be well informed about the potential risks. Young people experiencing psychiatric difficulties may be doubly vulnerable with regard to their capacity to understand these risks and participate in research (Spetie & Arnold, 2007). Thus, there are special considerations when carrying out pediatric clinical trials that involve mental health research (Shaddy, Denne, the Committee on Drugs, & the Committee on Pediatric Research, 2010).

Since the implementation of mandatory reporting requirements under section 801 of the FDAAA, investigators must also include a statement on informed consent forms for applicable clinical trials regarding the availability of clinical trial information on ClinicalTrials.gov. The degree to which this information is being shared with and understood by participants, including the extent to which it influences decisions to participate in clinical trials, is unknown.

Limitations

While the results described here provide a comprehensive review of the land-scape in the field of pediatric clinical trials for APs, there are some limitations to the methods. Data from clinical trial registries was gathered and analyzed as the best representative sample of clinical trials; however, it is likely that not all trials are registered, particularly in jurisdictions where there is no requirement to register, or if peer-reviewed publication is not an end goal. In addition, our study focused only on clinical trials including children and youth, aged 18 years or less, excluding trials that also involved adult participants. Our results are therefore understood in the context of child/adolescent-only trials and do not represent the full range of pediatric involvement in clinical trials.

RECOMMENDATIONS

Public outreach about the importance of clinical trials and the risks involved with off-label medication is essential to challenge the perception that research is not beneficial to the individual, and concurrently that using clinical practice is not harmful to society. There is also a need for greater education about the ethical standards that are applied to research, to reassure the public that while the overall aim of a clinical trial is scientific knowledge, and not individual benefit, the researchers have a duty to their participants to be respectful of their contribution and are concerned for their welfare. These efforts must then be followed up with ethically designed and relevant clinical trials in areas where off-label use is identified as a particular concern. Although there is a lot of variance in the types of trials, indications, outcome measures, and drugs used for AP research in children, a transparent reporting process allows for systematic reviews and a more robust evaluation of the evidence and informs future trial design, especially if used by all. The benefits of registering trials on a publically accessible source are numerous: (1) it allows people to find information on participation in research; (2) it meets ethical and scientific obligations to ensure that research contributes to the medical evidence base; (3) it promotes scientific integrity; and (4) it provides summary information for exploring ethical, legal, and scientific aspects of the clinical research enterprise, which informs an appropriate allocation of resources (Zarin et al., 2013).

Although the total number of registered clinical trials for APs is greater than expected, the generalizability of their findings for physicians may be limited given the large variety of treatment combinations and types of trials. The diversity of trial characteristics, however, likely reflects the real world experience of patients and the doctors who treat them. Psychiatric disorders are often co-morbid, and polypharmacy is not uncommon. In other areas of health research, such as childhood cancers, advancements in treatment have been made despite a wide range of cancers with varying etiologies and small numbers of patient participants. The success of the pediatric oncology field may provide a model of how to enable therapeutic efficacy within a complex landscape. Medical progress was supported in pediatric oncology through a widespread acceptance of clinical research in this area, and the majority of children diagnosed were subsequently enrolled in a trial (Bleyer, 1997). Should a similar research model be employed within the context of childhood mental illness? Here, questions of risk and willingness to take on risk may emerge. Clinical trials for cancer may be more acceptable to parents as the potential lifesaving benefit may more easily outweigh the risks of involvement in a clinical trial.

In our analysis, only a handful of trials included a behavioral intervention. The inclusion of non-pharmacological interventions in clinical trials, which are potentially less risky and to some a more acceptable form of treatment for a child, is recommended. Relevant research into a wide range of therapeutic interventions should be hypothesis driven and directed by the potential for long-term benefit to the child. Consider the suggestion that an increase of clinical trials in APs be matched by an increase in trials of non-psychoactive treatments, for example behavioral interventions for behavioral presentations (Ashcroft, Fraser, Kerr, & Ahmed, 2001). Including a non-pharmacological treatment arm in AP clinical trials would be ideal, although perhaps unfeasible in light of funding sources and motivations. In contrast, there is a growing body of evidence that preventative pharmacological intervention may be beneficial for psychosis; again, more research is required to clarify this (McGorry, Yung, & Phillips, 2001).

Off-label prescribing is widely recognized as necessary for optimal patient care (Beck & Azari, 1998). In the case of children, however, the systemic widespread application of adult information without consideration of its impact on children creates widespread concern. Not only are more AP clinical trials required, more relevant and comparable trials are needed. Sound hypothesis-based trials would target finite clinical trial resources to interventions that are most likely to be effective in improving outcomes for children and their families. The landscape of clinical trial research outlined here is promising, given that there is a relevant and diverse field of pediatric clinical trials for APs and that these trials may drive approval indications for pediatric AP use in the clinic. This momentum may provide benefits to children and the clinician's who prescribe AP's to them.

REFERENCES

Amara, S. G., Grillner, S., Insel, T., Nutt, D., & Tsumoto, T. (2011). Neuroscience in recession? *Nature Reviews Neuroscience, 12,* 297–302.

Arnold, L. E. (2001). Turn-of-the-century ethical issues in child psychiatric research. *Current Psychiatry Reports, 3,* 109–114.

Ashcroft, R., Fraser, B., Kerr, M., & Ahmed, Z. (2001). Are antipsychotic drugs the right treatment for challenging behaviour in learning disability? The place of a randomised trial. *Journal of Medical Ethics, 27,* 338–343.

Avard, D., Black, L., Samuel, J., Griener, G., & Knoppers, B. M. (2012). *Best practices for health research involving children and adolescents; genetic, pharmaceutical and longitudinal studies (3rd draft)*. Center of Genomics and Policy (CGP), Maternal Infant Child and Youth Research Network (MICYRN), Canada.

Ballentine, C. (1981). Taste of raspberries, taste of death. The 1937 elixir sulfanilamide incident. *FDA Consumer Magazine*, Food and Drug Administration (FDA) History, Retrieved from http://www.fda.gov/aboutfda/whatwedo/history/productregulation/sulfanilamidedisaster/default.htm, Accessed May 6.

Bavdekar, S. B. (2013). Pediatric clinical trials. *Perspectives in Clinical Research*, 4(1), 89–99.

Beck, J. M., & Azari, E. D. (1998). FDA, off-label use, and informed consent: Debunking myth and misconceptions. *Food and Drug Law Journal*, 53, 71–104.

Belmont Report. (1979). *The Belmont report: Ethical principles and guidelines for the protection of human subjects of research*. hhs.gov/ohrp/humansubjects/guidance/belmont.html, Retrieved 06.04.14.

Bleyer, W. A. (1997). The U.S. pediatric cancer clinical trials programmes: International implications and the way forward. *European Journal of Cancer*, 33(9), 1439–1447. http://dx.doi.org/10.1016/S0959-8049(97)00249-9, PMID 9337687.

Bourgeois, F. T., Murthy, S., & Mandl, K. D. (2010). Outcome reporting among drug trials registered in clinicaltrials.gov. *Annals of Internal Medicine*, 153, 158–166.

Caldwell, P., Murphy, S. B., Butow, P. N., & Craig, J. C. (2004). Clinical trials in children. *The Lancet*, 364, 803–811.

Campbell Alliance. (2005). The era of clinical trial registries: A white paper. Retrieved from, http://www.campbellalliance.com/articles/Final_Clinical_Trial_Registries_3-23-05.pdf.

Canadian Institutes of Health Research, Natural Sciences and Engineering Research Council of Canada, & Social Sciences and Humanities Research Council of Canada. (2010). *Tri-council policy statement: Ethical conduct for research involving humans*. Retrieved from, http://www.pre.ethics.gc.ca/pdf/eng/tcps2/TCPS_2_FINAL_Web.pdf. Accessed 05.05.14.

Canadian Mental Health Association. (n.d.). Fast facts about mental illness in youth. http://www.cmha.ca/media/fast-facts-about-mental-illness/#.VDtKq1fQ2-A, Retrieved 06.04.2014.

Canadian Paediatric Society, & Drug Therapy and Hazardous Substances Committee. (2011). Drug research and treatment for children in Canada: A challenge. *Paediatrics and Child Health*, 16(9), 560.

Chan, A., Krleza-Ieric, K., Schmid, I., & Altman, D. G. (2004). Outcome reporting bias in randomized trials funded by the Canadian Institutes of Health Research. *Canadian Medial Association Journal*, 171(7), 735–740. http://dx.doi.org/10.1503/cmaj.1041086.

Committee on Bioethics. (1995). Informed consent, parental permission, and assent in pediatric practice. *Pediatrics*, 95, 314.

ARVO-Editorial. (2006). ARVO statement on registering clinical trials. *Investigative Ophthalmology & Visual Science*, 47(1), 1–2.

European Medicines Agency. (2007). *EU regulation on pediatric regulation*. Retrieved from http://www.ema.europa.eu/ema/index.jsp?curl=pages/regulation/document_listing/document_listing_000068.jsp.

Evans, C. H. & Ildstad, S. T. (Eds.). (2001). *Small clinical trials, issues & challenges*. Washington, DC: National Academy Press.

FDA News & Events. (2012). *50 Years: The Kefauver-Harris amendments. Food and Drug Administration (FDA) News & Events*. Retrieved from http://www.fda.gov/drugs/newsevents/ucm320924.htm, Accessed 05.05.14.

FDAAA 801 Requirements. (n.d.). FDAAA 801 Requirements. Retrieved from https://clinicaltrials.gov/ct2/manage-recs/fdaaa, Accessed on 06.04.14.

Freedman, B. (1987). Equipoise and the ethics of clinical research. *New England Journal of Medicine*, 317, 141–145.

Friedman, L. M., Furberg, C. D., & DeMets, D. L. (1996). *Fundamentals of clinical trials* (3rd ed.). New York: Springer.

Hart, B., Lundh, A., & Bero, L. (2012). Effect of reporting bias on meta-analyses of drug trials: Reanalysis of meta-analyses. *British Medical Journal, 344*, d7202.

Hopewell, S., Loudon, K., Clarke, M. J., Oxman, A. D., & Dickersin, K. (2009). Publication bias in clinical trials due to statistical significance or direction of trial results. *Cochrane Database of Systematic Reviews* (1). http://dx.doi.org/10.1002/14651858.MR000006.pub3, Art. No.: MR000006.

ICMJE Editorial. (2004). Clinical trial registration: A statement from The International Committee of Medical Journal editors. *The New England Journal of Medicine, 351*(12), 1250–1251.

Jones, C. W., Handler, L., Crowell, K. E., Keil, L. G., Weaver, M. A., & Platts-Mills, T. F. (2013). Non-publication of large randomized clinical trials: Cross sectional analysis. *British Medical Journal, 347*, http://dx.doi.org/10.1136/bmj.f6104.

Jong, G. W., van der Anker, J., & Choonara, I. (2001). FDAMA's written request list: Medicines for children (Letter to the Editor). *The Lancet, 357*, 398.

Koelch, M., Schnoor, K., & Fegert, J. M. (2008). Ethical issues in psychopharmacology of children and adolescents. *Current Opinion in Psychiatry, 21*, 598–605.

Kumar, A., Datta, S. S., Wright, S. D., Furtado, V. A., & Russell, P. S. (2013). Atypical antipsychotics for psychosis in adolescents. *Cochrane Database of Systematic Reviews, 10*, http://dx.doi.org/10.1002/14651858.CD009582.pub2, Art. No.: CD009582.

Lee, K., Bacchetti, P., & Sim, I. (2008). Publication of clinical trials supporting successful new drug applications: A literature analysis. *PLoS Medicine, 5*, e191.

McGorry, P. D., Yung, A., & Phillips, L. (2001). Ethics and early intervention in psychosis: Keeping up the pace and staying in step. *Schizophrenia Research, 51*, 17–29.

Murthy, S., Mandl, K. D., & Bourgeois, F. (2013). Analysis of pediatric clinical drug trials for neuropsychiatric conditions. *Pediatrics, 131*(6), 1125–1131.

Pediatric Final Rule. (1998). Regulations requiring manufacturers to assess the safety and effectiveness of new drugs and biological products in pediatric patients; final rule, 63 Federal Register 66632; December 2, 1998.

Peterson, B., Hebert, P. C., MacDonald, N., Rosenfield, D., Stanbrook, M. B., & Flegel, K. (2011). Industry's neglect of prescribing information for children (Editorial). *Canadian Medical Association Journal, 183*(9), 994–995.

Piantadosi, S. (1997). *Clinical trials: A methodologic perspective*. Hoboken, NJ: Wiley-Interscience.

Prayle, A. P., Hurley, M. N., Smyth, A. R., Prayle, A. P., Hurley, M. N., & Smyth, A. R. (2011). Compliance with mandatory reporting of clinical trial results on clinical trials.gov: Cross sectional study. *British Medical Journal, 344*, http://dx.doi.org/10.1136/bmj.d7373.

Ross, J. S., Mulvey, G. K., Hines, E. M., Nissen, S. E., & Krumholz, H. M. (2009). Trial publication after registration in clinicaltrials.gov: A cross-sectional analysis. *PLoS Medicine, 6*(9), e1000144. http://dx.doi.org/10.1371/journal.pmed.1000144.

Schuster, D. P. & Powers, W. J. (Eds.). (2005). *Translational and experimental clinical research*. Philadelphia: Lippincott Williams & Wilkins.

Shaddy, R. E., Denne, S. C., Committee on Drugs, & Committee on Pediatric Research. (2010). Guidelines for the ethical conduct of studies to evaluate drugs in pediatric populations. *Pediatrics, 125*, 850. http://dx.doi.org/10.1542/peds.2010-0082.

Shirkey, H. (1999). Editorial comment: Therapeutic orphans. *Pediatrics, 104*, 583.

Song, F., Parekh, S., Hooper, L., Loke, Y. K., Ryder, J., Sutton, A. J., et al. (2010). Dissemination and publication of research findings: An updated review of related biases. *Health Technology Assessment, 14*, iii, ix-xi, 1-193.

Spetie, L., & Arnold, L. E. (2007). Ethical issues in child psychopharmacology research and practice: Emphasis on preschoolers. *Psychopharmacology*, *191*, 15–26.

Sugarman, J. (2002). Ethics in the design and conduct of clinical trials. *Epidemiologic Reviews*, *24*(1), 54–58.

Thall, P. F. (2008). A review of phase 2-3 clinical trial designs. *Lifetime Data Analysis*, *14*, 37–53. http://dx.doi.org/10.1007/s10985-007-9049-x.

Thaul, S. (2012). *FDA's authority to ensure that drugs prescribed to children are safe and effective. Congressional Research Service: Report for Congress*. Downloaded from http://fas.org/sgp/crs/misc/RL33986.pdf, Accessed 07.10.14.

U.S. Food and Drug Administration. (2002). *Best pharmaceuticals for children act*. Retrieved from http://bpca.nichd.nih.gov/about/Pages/Index.aspx.

Weimer, K., Gulewitsch, M. D., Schlarb, A. A., Schwille-Kiuntke, J., Klosterhalfen, S., & Enck, P. (2013). Placebo effects in children: A review. *Pediatric Research*, *74*(1), 96–102.

Wendler, D., Rackoff, J. E., Emanuel, E. J., & Grady, C. (2002). The ethics of paying for children's participation in research. *The Journal of Pediatrics*, *141*(2), 166–171.

WHO. (2007). *Better medicines for children*. Downloaded from www.who.int/gb/ebwha/pdf_files/WHA60/A60_R20-en.pdf.

Williams, K., Thomson, D., Seto, I., Contopoulos-Ioannidis, D. G., Ioannidis, J. P. A., Curtis, S., et al. (2012). Standard 6: Age groups for pediatric trials. *Pediatrics*, *129*, S153–S160. http://dx.doi.org/10.1542/peds.2012-0055I.

WMA (World Medical Association): Declaration of Helsinki. (2013). Retrieved from http://www.wma.net/en/30publications/10policies/b3/.

Zarin, D. A., Williams, R. J., Bergeris, A. M., Dobbins, H., Ide, N. C., Loane, R. F, Robbins, A. & Tse, T. (2013). ClinicalTrials.gov and related projects: Improving access to information about clinical trials; A report to the board of scientific counselors. Technical report TR-2013-001. Bethesda, Maryland: Lister Hill National Center for Biomedical Communications, US National Library of Medicine.

Chapter 6

Pathways to Overmedication and Polypharmacy: Case Examples from Adolescents with Fetal Alcohol Spectrum Disorders

Osman Ipsiroglu[*,†,‡], Mai Berger[*,‡], Tami Lin[*,‡], Dean Elbe[¶,§], Sylvia Stockler[‡,#], Bruce Carleton[‖]

[*]Sleep/Wake Behaviour Clinic & Research Lab, BC Children's Hospital, Division of Developmental Pediatrics, Department of Pediatrics, Faculty of Medicine, University of British Columbia, Vancouver, British Columbia, Canada
[†]Faculty of Science, Thompson Rivers University, Kamloops, British Columbia, Canada
[‡]Person Centered Medicine, Treatable Intellectual Disability Endeavour in British Columbia (TIDE BC), Vancouver, British Columbia, Canada
[¶]Faculty of Pharmaceutical Sciences, University of British Columbia, Vancouver, British Columbia, Canada
[§]Child & Adolescent Mental Health, BC Children's Hospital, Vancouver, British Columbia, Canada
[#]Division of Biochemical Diseases, Department of Pediatrics, Faculty of Medicine, University of British Columbia, Vancouver, British Columbia, Canada
[‖]BC Children's Hospital, Division of Translational Therapeutics, Department of Pediatrics, Child & Family Research Institute, University of British Columbia, Vancouver, British Columbia, Canada

INTRODUCTION

Overview

Prescription drugs are one of the most important clinical treatments. With the wide spectrum of pharmacologic therapies currently on the market, it can be difficult to select a drug most likely to benefit a specific patient. This is particularly difficult in children or youth with neurodevelopmental conditions due to the complex, heterogeneous, and multifactorial nature of their clinical presentations. Fetal alcohol spectrum disorders (FASDs) are the most common form of prenatally acquired brain injury and are due to prenatal substance exposure (PSE) and the deleterious effects of alcohol on the developing brain of the fetus (Clarren & Smith, 1978; Jones & Smith, 1973). The Public Health Agency of Canada (2005) estimates that FASDs affect 1% of the Canadian population.

The Science and Ethics of Antipsychotic Use in Children. http://dx.doi.org/10.1016/B978-0-12-800016-8.00006-4

Depending on the methodology and magnitude of studies, prevalence rates change; in the United States, 0.2-1.5 out of every 1000 live births are affected with an FASD (May et al., 2009). FASDs encompass a spectrum of diagnoses ranging from fetal alcohol syndrome, the severest form among FASDs, including growth deficiency or facial characteristics, to partial fetal alcohol syndrome and alcohol-related neurodevelopmental disorder, characterized by a range of neurological and behavioral impairments, and alcohol-related birth defects, which refers to defects in other organs, skeletal abnormalities, and vision and hearing problems (Chudley et al., 2005; Public Health Agency of Canada, 2005; Rasmussen, Andrew, Zwaigenbaum, & Tough, 2008).

In this chapter, we analyze prescription practices in adolescents with an FASD diagnosis, as this population is prone to multiple prescription medications (Chudley et al., 2005; O'Malley & Nanson, 2002; Paley & O'Connor, 2009). We present our experience and the understanding taken from our collaborative clinical and pharmaceutical work to demonstrate how chronic sleep problems in children and youth with complex neurodevelopmental conditions (such as FASDs) can become the gateway to treatments with multiple, off-label, and concurrent pharmaceutical medications over time. We refer to this practice as *polypharmacy*.

Our finding is that tackling sleep problems as a primary treatment target starting at a young age reduces the trend to overmedication and polypharmacy and improves outcomes in adolescents with neurodevelopmental conditions and challenging day and nighttime behaviors. The results from our case series analysis represent a first step toward practice-based evidence. We believe that our finding and recommendations can be applied within the broader context of children and youth who receive treatment with psychotropic medications for a variety of mental health conditions. We suggest that in children with neurodevelopmental disorders the use of medications such as antipsychotics and stimulants to treat challenging/disruptive daytime behaviors can be reduced or even eliminated after treating underlying sleep disorders. Our aim is to highlight how an alternative intervention approach may be used to stop the trend toward overmedication of children, which leads to polypharmacy at adolescent age. In other words, our aim is to lessen the need for pharmacological interventions in patients suffering from neurodevelopmental conditions and comorbid behavioral presentations such as conduct disorder or attention-deficit/hyperactivity disorder (ADHD). We do not suggest that pharmaceutical treatment is unnecessary; on the contrary, many individuals with neurodevelopmental conditions will benefit better from medication after identifying and targeting underlying sleep problems.

Sleep problems in children with neurodevelopmental conditions: The importance of sleep is well documented with regard to cognition, emotional and physical resilience, and wellbeing or quality of life. In adults, addressing sleep problems has a long tradition, originating in ancient cultures (Brunt & Steger, 2008). Sleep problems have been recognized as a key symptom of neurodevelopmental conditions (Bruni & Novelli, 2010; Wiggs & Stores, 1996; Wiggs, 2001; Zucconi & Bruni, 2001). However, in spite of their documented negative impacts on psychomotor development and cognitive and behavioral functioning (Jan, Bax, Owens, Ipsiroglu, & Wasdell, 2012), sleep problems are not systematically integrated into current assessment and treatment practice. Lack of training and assessment tools as well as a siloed subspecialist approach hinder the recognition of sleep problems as significant contributors to illness and reduced quality of life (Ipsiroglu, McKellin, Carey, & Loock, 2013; Jan et al., 2008). Furthermore, the cause of an underlying sleep problem is difficult to identify, as nighttime behaviors are not accessible to direct clinical observation outside a sleep lab or hospital-based environment.

In our clinical work, we have observed a high prevalence of Willis Ekbom disease (WED; formerly known as restless legs syndrome) presentations in children and adolescents with an FASD and/or PSE diagnosis (Ipsiroglu et al., 2013). WED is an example of a treatable neurologic disorder that impacts sleep and is underdiagnosed in children. WED is prevalent in 5-10% of the general population, and is associated with major sleep problems in 2-3% adults (Allen et al., 2005). Prevalence rates of WED that impacts sleep are similar in children (Picchietti et al., 2007). The challenge is that a WED diagnosis is based on the patient's subjective expression of discomfort (Picchietti et al., 2011) and there are currently no diagnostic protocols allowing for recognition of WED in children who are unable to express themselves (Picchietti et al., 2013). As WED is associated with both night- and daytime restlessness, it is often misdiagnosed as ADHD (Picchietti, 2013; Walters et al., 2008). Treatment with typical ADHD medications (psychostimulants) often results in behavioral or other adverse effects, perpetuating the challenging sleep and daytime behaviors. Accurate diagnosis of WED is of clinical relevance as it allows for disease-specific treatment options such as iron supplementation, levodopa, and gabapentin (Magnus, 1999; Picchietti, 2013; Robinson & Malow, 2012).

Sleep problems are a key symptom of individuals with FASDs (Steinhausen & Spohr, 1998; Streissguth, Barr, Kogan, & Bookstein, 1996), but due to overriding behavioral comorbidities they often remain undiagnosed (Ipsiroglu et al., 2013; Jan et al., 2010). Thus, knowledge about the phenotype of FASD-related sleep problems is limited. In addition to our work (Ipsiroglu et al., 2013), the association between sleep problems and daytime behaviors has been presented in only two other studies: (1) Chen, Olson, Picciano, Starr, and Owens (2012) showed significant sleep problems in a population with FASD referred for behavioral intervention; and (2) Wengel, Hanlon-Dearman, and Fjelsted (2011) demonstrated that unidentified sensory processing abnormalities contribute to behavioral problems and insomnia (falling asleep, sleep maintenance problems) in FASD patients.

FASDs, overmedication, and polypharmacy: Children with an FASD represent one of the most vulnerable populations in terms of psychotropic drug prescription. Their birth mothers, and even foster parents, face social stigma associated with the condition because it is the result of potentially preventable toxic alcohol exposure during pregnancy (Hill, Hegemier, & Tennyson, 1989; Oldani, 2009; Ryan & Ferguson, 2006). The social stigma might lead caregivers to seek out medications and physicians to prescribe them to attenuate the impact that FASDs have on cognitive functioning and behavior (Oldani, 2009). The functioning and behaviors of children with an FASD typically resembles ADHD; however, research has only partial response to pharmacologic treatments aimed at addressing ADHD symptoms (Coles, 2001; Rasmussen et al., 2008). Literature suggests that, in complex clinical presentations, multiple medications should be trialed in order to find the right treatment (O'Malley, 1997; O'Malley, Koplin, & Dohner, 2000; O'Malley & Nanson, 2002; O'Malley & Streissguth, 2005; Wilens, Spencer, Biederman, Wozniak, & Connor, 1995). At our follow-up clinic, observation has shown a high prevalence of behavioral adverse drug reactions (ADRs) upon treatment of ADHD-like behaviors with stimulants and antipsychotics, leading to a cascade of additional diagnoses (interpreted as FASD comorbidities) and treatments, and eventual breakdown in family situations resulting in placements as depicted by the case vignette on p. 138.

MEDICATION HISTORY IN 17 CHILDREN WITH AN FASD AND SLEEP PROBLEMS

We retrospectively analyzed medical records to capture the medication history of adolescents with FASDs/PSE who had been assessed for their challenging/disruptive sleep/wake behaviors at our clinic. We were mainly interested in (1) the drugs used and the order in which they were prescribed, and (2) the age of the patient at the time of the first prescription.

During the time period between 2010 and 2014, 20 pediatric patients with an FASD or PSE diagnosis above the age of 10 had been referred to our clinic by community pediatricians for assessment of their sleep problems. In 17 patients (age range: 10-17 years, median age: 13 years) we created a pharmacotherapy timeline (see Figure 6.1 for an example). Patients included in our analysis had the following sleep/wake behaviors and neurodevelopmental conditions.

- All 17 patients fulfilled the diagnostic criteria for WED and/or familial WED and showed evidence for disordered circadian rhythm sleep disorders caused by insomnia and a nonrestorative sleep quality.
- Seventeen (100%) patients had falling asleep problems; 10 patients (59%) had sleep maintenance problems, and 1 had early morning awakenings.
- Eleven (65%) patients also had clinical evidence of sleep-disordered breathing and 5 (29%) had regular washroom awakenings over the night.
- Fourteen (82%) patients showed excessive daytime behaviors (sleepiness and/or hyperactive-like behaviors to fight fatigue/sleepiness) and eight (47%) were increasingly fidgety toward the evening and/or at bedtime.

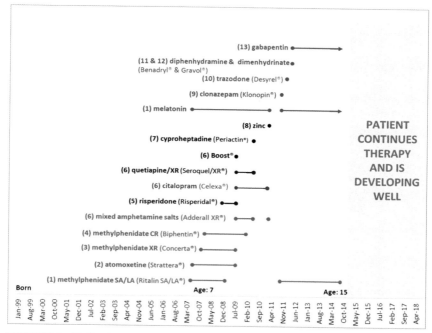

FIGURE 6.1 Medication use details for case vignette. This figure depicts the medication use order and time courses for the case vignette presented on p. 138. Medications for ADHD-like behaviors are depicted in red; atypical antipsychotics and SSRIs are depicted in blue and purple, respectively; supplements are depicted in black; and medications targeting sleep are depicted in green. The numbers preceding the medications represent the chronological order of each medication. Medications that are ongoing (not discontinued) are depicted with an arrow. Abbreviations: SA, short-acting; LA, long-acting; XR, extended release; CR, controlled release.

- Sixteen patients (94%) also presented with one or more coexisting neurodevelopmental conditions, such as autism spectrum disorder ($n=2$; 12%), ADHD ($n=15$; 88%), or mental health disorders, such as anxiety disorders ($n=11$; 65%), oppositional defiant disorder ($n=7$; 41%), or mood disorders ($n=6$; 35%).

Table 6.1 gives a detailed overview of the sleep/wake-behavior assessment results, neurodevelopmental conditions, and comorbidities.

The medication history of patients in our sample included the following highlights (see Table 6.2 for further details).

- In total, 120 medication trials were prescribed across the 17 patients, most of them in sequential order over a period of time. There was only one medication-naive patient who was assessed for sleep/wake-problems (at the age of 13).
- The maximum number of medication trials prescribed to a patient over the time was 21. This patient was 14 years old at the time of our assessment and was diagnosed with an FASD and PSE, mood disorder, moderate to severe ADHD, and anxiety.

TABLE 6.1 Patient Demographics and Day/Nighttime Clinical Presentation in Pediatric Patients with FASDs and/or PSE

Patients with an FASD/ PSE Diagnosis and Associated Medical Conditions	Diagnoses	Percentage of Patients (%)
Sleep disorders	Excessive daytime behaviors (sleepiness and/or hyperactive-like behaviors to fight fatigue/sleepiness)	82
	Circadian rhythm sleep disorder (CRSD)	100[a]
	Sleep disordered breathing (SDB)	65[b]
	Periodic limb movements (PLM)	53
	Insomnia	100
	Parasomnias	76
Neurodevelopmental conditions	Attention-deficit hyperactivity disorder (ADHD)	88
	Autism spectrum disorder (ASD)	12[c]
Mental health or psychiatric comorbidities	Anxiety disorder	65
	Oppositional defiant disorder (ODD)	41
	Mood disorder	35
	Reactive attachment disorder (RAD)	35
	Obsessive-compulsive disorder (OCD)	11
Neurologic comorbidities	Willis Ekbom disease (WED)	100[d]
	Sensory processing abnormalities (SPAs)	94[e]

All patients presented FASDs and/or PSE, as well as sleep disorders. A total of 94% were diagnosed with other neurodevelopmental conditions besides FASDs and PSE, the most common being attention-deficit/hyperactivity disorder (ADHD, 88%). There was also a high incidence of psychiatric disorders such as anxiety disorder (65%) and oppositional defiant disorder (ODD, 41%).
a 14/17 patients had confirmed CRSD; 3/17 patients had highly suspected CRSD.
b 8/11 patients had confirmed SDB; 3/11 patients had suspected SDB.
c 2/17 patients had suspected ASD due to their clinical presentation, but the diagnosis was not confirmed after formal assessment.
d 11/17 patients had confirmed WED; 6/17 patients had suspected WED.
e 16/17 patients had confirmed SPAs; 1/17 patients had suspected SPAs.

- All patients except the medication-naive patient were treated with medications for their sleep problems (94%; in total, 39 medication trials with prescription medications or over-the-counter sleep medications). Sleep medications topped the prescription list when we further analyzed median and maximum number of medications prescribed or bought over-the-counter.

TABLE 6.2 Prescription and Medication Practices in Pediatric Patients with FASDs and/or PSE

N=17 Mean Age: 13 years Median Age: 13 years Range: 10–17 years	All Medications	Sleep Medication Clonazepam, Clonidine, Chlorpromazine[a], Dimenhydrinate, Diphenhydramine, Lorazepam, Melatonin, Quetiapine[b], Trazodone	ADHD Medication Atomoxetine, Methylphenidate (Biphentin®, Concerta®, Ritalin®), Dextroamphetamine, Guanfacine, Lisdexamfetamine, Mixed Amphetamine Salts	Second-generation Antipsychotics (Daytime) Aripiprazole, Olanzapine, Quetiapine[a], Risperidone	SSRI Citalopram, Fluoxetine, Paroxetine, Sertraline	Anticonvulsants Lamotrigine, Topiramate, Sodium Valproate, Valproic Acid	Other[b] Docusate, Gabapentin, Imipramine, Iron, Lithium, Propranolol
Medication categories							
% Patients prescribed medication	94%	94%	76%	59%	47%	24%	29%
Number of medications per patient (mean/median)[c]	7.1/6	2.5/2	1.71/1	1.18/1	0.70/1	0.47/0	0.47/0
Max/min number of medication prescribed per patient per drug class	21/0	5/0	5/0	4/0	2/0	4/0	2/0

(Continued)

TABLE 6.2 Prescription and Medication Practices in Pediatric Patients with FASDs and/or PSE—cont'd

N=17 Mean Age: 13 years Median Age: 13 years Range: 10-17 years	All Medications	Sleep Medication	ADHD Medication	Second-generation Antipsychotics (Daytime)	SSRI	Anticonvulsants	Other[b]
Most common medications		Clonazepam, Clonidine, Chlorpromazine[a], Dimenhydrinate, DiphenhydramIne, Lorazepam, Melatonin, Quetiapine[b], Trazodone	Atomoxetine, Methylphenidate (Biphentin®, Concerta®, Ritalin®), Dextroamphetamine, Guanfacine, Lisdexamfetamine, Mixed Amphetamine Salts	Aripiprazole, Olanzapine, Quetiapine[a], Risperidone	Citalopram, Fluoxetine, Paroxetine, Sertraline	Lamotrigine, Topiramate, Sodium Valproate, Valproic Acid	Docusate, Gabapentin, Imipramine, Iron, Lithium, Propranolol
Most commonly prescribed medication per drug class	Melatonin	Melatonin	Concerta®, dextroamphetamine	Risperidone	Fluoxetine	Lamotrigine, topiramate, valproic acid	Iron
% Patients prescribed most common medications per drug class (or category)[d]	35%	35%	41%	40%	50%	75%	38%

First medication prescription							
% First medication prescribed	N/A	41%	41%	0%[e]	6%[f]	0%	0%
Mean age at first prescription overall	6.8 years	7.9 years	7.8 years	6 years	5 years	N/A	N/A
Youngest age at first prescription overall	2.5 years	3 years	2.5 years	5 years	5 years	N/A	N/A
Age at first prescription per drug class (mean/median)	N/A	8.4/7 years	7.5/7	9.6/8 years	9/9 years	N/A	N/A

Sleep medications were the most commonly prescribed drugs of this cohort, and made up the majority of the first prescribed medications (94%). ADHD medications were shown to be prescribed at the youngest age overall (2.5 years), while SSRIs were prescribed at the youngest mean age at first prescription (5 years).
a This medication is regarded as an antipsychotic; however, chlorpromazine was used in 2 patients at low dosages for targeting sleep problems.
b Quetiapine was used to target both sleep and daytime behaviors; this was taken into account by categorizing it in either the Sleep Medication or Second-Generation Antipsychotics (daytime) column, according to its target symptom.
c Prescribed prior to assessment at the Sleep/Wake Behavior Clinic.
d This number is an approximation and was calculated from available documentation.
e Twelve percent of patients were first prescribed quetiapine to target sleep problems and not daytime behaviors.
f One patient was prescribed fluoxetine as his first medication.

- ADHD mediations were most commonly prescribed for daytime behaviors (76%; in total 29 prescription trials) followed by first- and second-generation antipsychotics (59%; in total 20 prescription trials), selective serotonin reuptake inhibitors (SSRIs) (47%; in total 12 prescription trials), and anticonvulsants (24%; in total 8 prescription trials) for challenging/disruptive daytime behaviors.
- Over one-third of patients were also treated with prescription and over-the-counter medications categorized as others (including iron supplements, lorazepam, chlorpromazine, propranolol, lithium, imipramine, docusate, and gabapentin, or 35%; in total 12 prescriptions). For example, seven (41%) patients received over-the-counter melatonin for their underlying sleep problems as their first medication, either by the recommendation of their physician or by their own discretion. The youngest patient was 3 years old when melatonin was first given.
- Seven (41%) patients were prescribed their first medication at age 5 years or younger.
- Seven (41%) patients were first prescribed psychostimulants and ADHD medications to target hyperactive-like daytime presentations. The youngest patient was 2.5 years of age when methylphenidate was first prescribed; this patient did not tolerate methylphenidate, and after 1 week the medication was changed to dextroamphetamine, which was also not tolerated and had to be stopped.
- Two patients (12%) received second-generation antipsychotics, prescribed for sleep problems, as the first medication; the youngest patient was 5 years old at the time of the first prescription.
- One patient (6%) received an SSRI as the first medication at the age of 5 years.

Table 6.2 gives an overview of the prescription medications, including the most common medications and first prescription medication, given to patients with an FASD and/or PSE diagnosis.

CASE VIGNETTE DEMONSTRATING INTERACTIONS BETWEEN SLEEP PROBLEMS, WED, AND ADRS

A 12-year-old female patient with an FASD diagnosis presented at the Sleep/ Wake-Behaviour Clinic of British Columbia Children's Hospital (Department of Pediatrics; University of British Columbia, Vancouver, Canada) with insomnia, specifically falling asleep and sleep maintenance problems. In the medical records, sleep problems were noted at age 6, and are described as associated with starting medications; however, in the disease narrative, sleep problems (insomnia and restless sleep) were mentioned as early as 19 months. Concerns of speech delay, behavioral control, and social interaction were initially raised in kindergarten (age 5 years), and the probability of ASD was noted and eventually ruled out (by age 7 years). At age 7, the patient was diagnosed with ADHD and partial FAS; at the age of 9 years comorbid anxiety, reactive attachment disorder, and mixed receptive/expressive language disorders were diagnosed. Additionally, the patient was described to have obsessive-compulsive and oppositional defiant-like behaviors at the age of 11.

A total of 11 psychotropic medications, several central nervous system stimulants and second-generation antipsychotics, were trialed starting shortly after the initial ADHD diagnosis, between the ages of 7 and 12 years, with little or no success. The neurologic/behavioral/metabolic ADRs to prescribed medications contributed to two emergency admissions to psychiatry. She was 7 years old when first prescribed methylphenidate (Ritalin®), which was ineffective and in fact exacerbated her oppositional behavior. She was simultaneously trialed on atomoxetine and again methylphenidate (Concerta®), both of which were "unable to alleviate symptoms of inattention, hyperactivity, and impulsivity" and also aggravated her sleep difficulties. She was hospitalized at age 9 for a behavioral outburst. At the hospital, she was switched from her previous three ADHD medications to mixed amphetamine salts (Adderall XR®). This proved unsuccessful and concerns regarding "poor appetite and suppression of normal spontaneity and enthusiasm" were raised. At 20 mg of mixed amphetamine salts, she experienced tachycardia. Risperidone was prescribed and proved to be ineffective, wherein her oppositional and disinhibited behavior increased. In addition, she experienced marked weight loss and appetite suppression from stimulant medication ("while [it is suspected that] her prenatal alcohol exposure is part of the picture, likely her stimulant medications are making things worse"), and was prescribed appetite stimulants such as cyproheptadine as a result.

For falling asleep problems, the patient was medicated with melatonin, which "did not help and induced parasomnias." Parasomnias are sleep disorders that present as movements (sleep walking), behaviors (sleep talking or night terrors), perceptions and dreams (hypnagogic hallucinations, as in the case of our patient) while falling asleep and/or between sleep stages (International Classification of Sleep Disorders, 2005). In consequence, she was prescribed quetiapine, which caused lipid abnormalities (high low-density lipoprotein). We reference one of her previous physicians, who described her as "one of the sickest children [she] had ever seen."

This case vignette has been visualized with a Life Trajectory Chart (Figure 6.2), depicting the effects of the medication on diagnoses and life events, such as the eventual family breakdown and placement in a group home.

Improvement of her challenging behaviors occurred after diagnosis of her underlying familial neurological condition, WED, and addressing the WED-related discomfort and sequelae (insomnia and restless sleep) with gabapentin at the age of 12. Improvements in her clinical presentation were as follows: (1) amount of sleep increased; (2) her sleep became restful and clinically more restorative as the number of her counted awakenings overnight decreased from approximately thirteen to zero; and (3) after a few months of therapy with

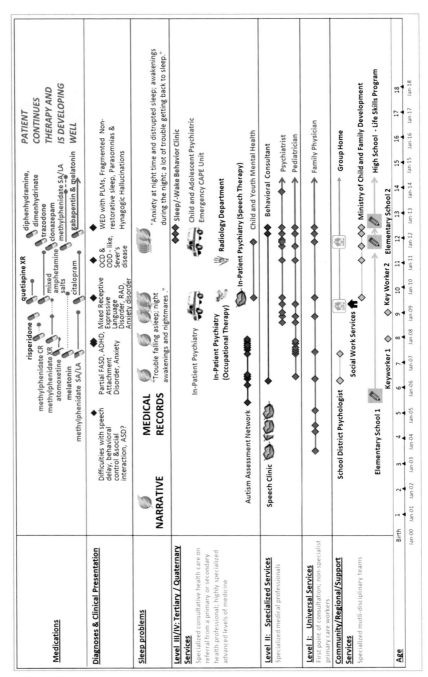

FIGURE 6.2   Cont'd

gabapentin (Magnus, 1999; Picchietti, 2013; Robinson & Malow, 2012), her anxiety decreased and she began to be able to sleep alone. In follow-up, it was retrospectively recognized that her anxiety was caused by hypnagogic hallucinations (occurring at transition from wakefulness to sleep). After 18 months of treatment, teachers described the patient as "resilient," she was able to advance in her math class from grade 3 to grade 7, and she could be sent to school alone on public transportation as she no longer required one-to-one supervision.

Retrospective analysis reveals that the patient's sleep problems were evident at early toddler age, but the clinical focus was placed on her challenging/disruptive daytime behaviors. Sleep problems, caused by her underlying familial WED condition, were clinically ignored. At her current age of 15 years, the patient is only taking gabapentin and prefers not to use psychostimulants to address her daytime ADHD-like behaviors as she associates these medications with nightmares.

DISCUSSION

Internationally, there is increasing concern regarding the prescription of psychotropic drugs to children. In 2012, Canada had the highest prescription rates for psychostimulants and antipsychotic medications for children in a multijurisdictional comparative study (Zhang et al., 2013). Complementing the recommendations of the Canadian Alliance for Monitoring Effectiveness and Safety of Antipsychotics in Children and the position statement released by the Canadian Paediatric Society, there are applicable prescription guidelines for children and adolescents (Pringsheim, Doja, Belanger, Patten, & CAMESA guideline group, 2011; Pringsheim, Panagiotopoulos, Davidson, Ho, & CAMESA guideline group, 2011). These guidelines emphasize the importance of initial evaluation and ongoing monitoring, limiting concurrent prescriptions, careful selection of first-line interventions, and adherence to evidence-based applications.

FIGURE 6.2 Life-trajectory graph for case vignette. Case vignette shows impact of missed sleep problems visualized on a life-trajectory graph. The patient presented with chronic SPs since very early childhood caused by WED, which had been (mis)labeled as attention-deficit hyperactivity disorder (ADHD), and was diagnosed with multiple mental health comorbidities (delays noted at age 5; fetal alcohol spectrum disorder and ADHD diagnosed at age 7; anxiety, attachment, and language disorders at age 9). In the medical records, sleep problems were noted at age 6 and described as associated with starting medications. However, in the caregiver narrative, sleep problems were mentioned as early as 19 months. She was treated for challenging/disruptive daytime behaviors with 11 prescription medications in various combinations, including hypnotics, stimulants, antipsychotics, antidepressants, and antiseizure and blood pressure medications, and up to 11 medications labeled as "food-supplements." The patient experienced several severe adverse drug reactions, with emergency admissions to pediatric or mental health facilities and a significantly impacted family ecology. Improvement of her challenging/disruptive behaviors occurred after diagnosis of the familial Willis Ekbom disease (WED) and treatment of WED-related discomfort with neuropathic pain medication. Abbreviations: SA, short-acting; LA, long-acting; XR, extended release; CR, controlled release.

Why haven't these guidelines been applied? Why are there still such high prescription rates?

Children with neurodevelopmental conditions and concurrent sleep problems are at particularly high likelihood for psychotropic drug prescriptions because of the intertwined relationship between their challenging day- and nighttime behaviors. As we were analyzing the medical histories of patients referred to our sleep/wake-behaviour clinic, it was evident that sleep problems were a prominent concern in all cases. Prior to referral, patient sleep problems (mainly insomnia) had already been targeted with melatonin, which topped the list of medications. Melatonin, clonidine, clonazepam, antihistamines, quetiapine, and trazodone all addressed insomnia but insufficiently, accounting for the number of different medication trials; thus, medications targeting sleep led the prescription list when we further analyzed median and maximum number of medications bought over-the-counter or prescribed.

Medications targeting ADHD had the first ranking among the medications prescribed for daytime behaviors, making up more than three-fourths of the patient prescriptions, followed by antipsychotics at almost two-thirds of the patient prescriptions. Second-generation antipsychotics were the most common antipsychotic class prescribed for the patient cohort. Only two patients were taking the first-generation antipsychotic chlorpromazine. Approximately one-half of the patients were taking SSRIs.

In our recent work, which was based on parent and healthcare professional descriptions and analyses of 27 child and youth patient histories, we conjectured that parents probably reported sleep problems during clinical assessments and, due to missing assessment tools, lack of training, and insufficient infrastructure, not followed up further (Ipsiroglu et al., 2013). Daytime-focused medication cascades did not improve the sleep problem and may have even aggravated the underlying condition. Therefore, the sequelae of medication cascades were a principle cause for eventual referral of patients to our clinic following an odyssey of assessments and treatment trials, as in the presented case vignette. The in-depth analysis of prescription strategies in the presented 17 patient histories of adolescents (defined here as children older than 10 years) and the case vignette demonstrate the dimension of this sleep-perspective-based conclusion for the first time. As shown, diagnosis and treatment cascades can be triggered if sleep problems are missed in the assessment of wake behaviors, and in consequence iatrogenic harm can occur.

WED and WED-like presentations deserve special attention as they manifest with both restless daytime behaviors mimicking ADHD and with restless night and sleep behaviors mimicking behavioral insomnia; together they resemble challenging/disruptive (externalizing) behaviors which justify prescription strategies exceeding current best practice guidelines (Canadian CADDRA Guidelines, 2011). Diagnosis of WED is based on subjective symptoms reported by the patient and, in the absence of a disease-specific biomarker, diagnosis of WED is challenging, particularly in children. Sensory discomfort and a shifted pain threshold, which is mostly associated with the typical motor hyperactivity, exacerbate abnormal behaviors. We hypothesize that there are two likely causes for difficulties with expressing subjective suffering in children. One is simply that they are too young or do not have the language capacity. The second one is that sensory processing abnormalities start at an early age and a reference point, which enables appropriate realization and description of sensations, is missing. In fact, 82% of the patients from the case series had sensory processing abnormalities. The Wengel et al.'s study (2011) supports our explanation and suggests a more in-depth explorative and observational assessment strategy, as recommended by the International WED Study Group (Picchietti et al., 2013). The recently published description of early onset familial WED (Allen et al., 2014; Tilma, Tilma, Norregaard, & Ostergaard, 2013) also supports the need for a more in-depth explorative and observational assessment strategy and additional criteria, such as assessment of parents and other family members, before focusing exclusively on daytime behaviors. In our assessments, we have been using (in cases where it is possible) a positive family history and signs of involuntary movements in a clinically adapted version of the suggested immobilization test (Michaud, 2006) in the child and the affected parent to establish the diagnosis.

As demonstrated in the case vignette, patients with WED can have severe adverse reactions to psychostimulants and/or antipsychotics treating neurological adverse effects, presenting as challenging/disruptive behaviors, for which additional stimulants and/or antipsychotics may trigger new symptoms and act as a catch-22, leading to further deterioration. In our case study, after treating WED with gabapentin, the patient's clinical presentation and life trajectory changed. Both her sleep problems and excessive daytime behaviors, including ADHD-like presentation and anxiety, improved. While her anxiety as well as her need for one-to-one supervision had been exclusively associated with pre-natal alcohol-related injury, the observed behavioral and mental health changes were very surprising for all care team members, who were convinced that the patient's behaviors were caused by prenatal alcohol exposure and its impacts on the developing brain. This transformation in clinical presentation highlights to what degree WED had aggravated, and even possibly caused, the mental health comorbidities, and that treatment with sleep helped her brain recover to a novel degree, perceived by the care team as unexpected.

Prescription Strategies and Challenges

The analysis of the 17 patients' first medications reveals two patterns in prescription strategies: (1) targeting sleep problems with melatonin, second-generation antipsychotics, and/or a combination of both (10/17; 59%); and (2) targeting hyperactive-like daytime behaviors with a psychostimulant (7/17; 41%).

The challenge with melatonin. Melatonin was trialed in all patients, excluding the one medication-naive patient, and was partly efficient in 14/17 (82%) cases for sleep initiation, but not for sleep maintenance. Since 2004, in Canada, melatonin has been sold over the counter as a licensed natural health product, with some review of safety and efficacy, while it is a prescription medication in most European countries. In this case series, melatonin dosages of up to 30 mg/day were applied, and in some cases medication was started already at very young age (3 years). Melatonin is a zeitgeber (an external cue to entrain circadian rhythms), but not a sedative. If given unselectively, aspects of the individual patient's sleep problems such as obstructive sleep apnea/hypopnea, sensory discomfort in WED, periodic limb movements during sleep, and other potential reasons for sleep problems such as pain, hunger, gastrointestinal discomfort (in children with nighttime G-tube feeding) may not be tackled and time to find the right treatment is lost. This might be the reason for contradicting literature, which praises and criticizes the effects of melatonin from various viewpoints (Buscemi & Witmans, 2006; Gringras et al., 2012; Jan et al., 2008, 2012). Our data show that in the absence of a sleep/wake behavior assessment and follow-up, melatonin is a starter drug in children with neurodevelopmental conditions (e.g., melatonin was first used in 41% of the 17 cases reported here) and sleep problems, and significantly contributes to the medication cascade.

The challenge with psychostimulants/ADHD medications. Children with FASD are diagnosed with ADHD six times more frequently than those without an FASD diagnosis (Rasmussen et al., 2010; Streissguth et al., 1996). Despite indications that the complexity of behavioral problems in this population cannot be explained by an ADHD-related pathophysiology alone (Coles, 2001; LaFrance et al., 2014), and despite variable responses to medications (e.g., lack of therapeutic response and/or ADRs) (Doig, McLennan, & Gibbard, 2008; O'Malley & Nanson, 2002; Rowles & Findling, 2010), ADHD-like symptoms are a frequent target for pharmacological interventions with psychostimulants. Indeed, 88% of our cohort presented with the comorbid condition ADHD. One patient from our cohort was a boy who was diagnosed with ADHD at age 2.5 years and was immediately trialed with two stimulants (methylphenidate and dextroamphetamine, each for approximately 1 week), with major behavioral ADRs. This case and another case seen at our clinic, where more than two psychostimulants had been prescribed at a time, demonstrate how desperate the parents and the prescribing physician were to find a solution for challenging/disruptive hyperactive behaviors (at that time in BC a sleep clinic investigating sleep/wake behaviors was not yet established). Guidelines for prescribing ADHD drugs suggest they not be administered until the patient is at least 4 years of age (Aagaard & Hansen, 2011; Canadian CADDRA Guidelines, 2011; Centers for Disease Control and Prevention, 2013; Wolraich et al., 2011). Furthermore, our data reveal that 41% of the cohort was prescribed a stimulant as the first medication, and that 38% were prescribed stimulants before the age of 6 years. Despite the fact that there are insufficient long-term studies and a lack of information on the effects of ADHD medication combinations, the American Academy of Pediatrics has expanded the age range for ADHD diagnosis in children to as young as 4 years (Wolraich et al., 2011). As a consequence, we may see treatment with psychopharmacology at even earlier ages become more commonplace in the near future.

Stepping back and observing from the viewpoint of a medical anthropologist (Oldani, 2009), it seems that prescription of ADHD medications, despite the lack of confidence in positive medication effects, became a strategy of action for relieving all involved parties. Children with restless daytime behaviors deserve particular attention and nonrestorative sleep quality as a reason for hyperactive-like behaviors to fight daytime fatigue/sleepiness needs to be ruled out prior to prescription of a psychostimulant. Most likely the high number of ADHD diagnoses (82% of all adolescents) is incorrect. Therefore, a reevaluation of all ADHD diagnoses becomes necessary. This hypothesis is further supported by the fact that none of the WED or Willis Ekbom-like presentations (which also resemble ADHD) had been diagnosed before the ADHD diagnosis. Figure 6.3 gives an overview of our understanding of how sleep problems affect day- and nighttime behavior presentations.

The Challenge with Second-Generation Antipsychotics. As described above, clinical circumstances in which there has been little or no therapeutic success often lead to deviations from guidelines and common prescription practices, such as prescribing atypical antipsychotics to children younger than 6 years, generally not recommended. Recent studies show that the rate of prescribing in children has been growing at a substantial rate (Findling et al., 2011; Ronsley et al., 2013; Therapeutics Initiative, 2009). In our population, almost 60% had been prescribed a second-generation antipsychotic at some time over their life trajectory, and almost one-half of the patients were prescribed an SSRI. These drugs were used in children as young as 6 and 5 years, respectively. In addition to ADHD, our cohort presented with a high comorbidity of psychiatric disorders, such as anxiety disorder (65%) and oppositional defiant disorder

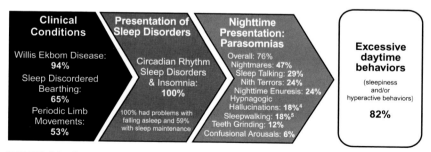

FIGURE 6.3   Impact of sleep problems on day/nighttime presentations (mean age: 13 years; median age: 13 years; range: 10-17 years). This figure depicts the complex interactions between challenging day- and nighttime presentations. Disorders such as Willis Ekbom disease (WED) and sleep disordered breathing (SDB) present with insomnia and contribute to circadian rhythm sleep disorders as well as to excessive daytime behaviors (sleepiness and/or hyperactive-like presentation). These in turn trigger arousal disorders such as parasomnias with a variety of presentations and result in excessive daytime behaviors.

(41%), a finding that has been consistently noted in the literature (Hellemans, Sliwowska, Verma, & Weinberg, 2010; O'Connor & Paley, 2009). However, the case vignette shows that anxiety, which prevented our patient from being able to sleep alone, was caused by sleep deprivation triggering hypnagogic hallucinations. Hypnagogic hallucinations belong to the sleep disorder category of parasomnias and, like all other parasomnias, are triggered by sleep deprivation, medications, and irregular sleep schedules. Treatment of WED enabled the patient to fall asleep and achieve a "good night's sleep" (restorative sleep), resulting in cessation of the hypnagogic hallucinations, and, over time, her anxiety also disappeared.

ADRs from second-generation antipsychotics, such as the ones described in our case vignette, have been well documented. Moreover, increasing numbers of children may be receiving antipsychotic or antidepressant medications for reasons not supported by scientific evidence, many without licensed approval (Findling et al., 2011; O'Connor & Paley, 2009) or off-evidence use (see Chapter 3). The Canadian Alliance for Monitoring Effectiveness and Safety of Antipsychotics in Children (CAMESA) guidelines aim to frame this discussion of how antipsychotic medication in pediatric patients should be managed (Ho et al., 2011; Pringsheim, Doja, et al., 2011; Pringsheim, Panagiotopoulos, et al., 2011).

The Challenge of Behavioral ADRs. "An adverse drug reaction is unwanted or harmful reaction experienced after the administration of a drug or combination of drugs under normal conditions of use and suspected to be related to the drug" (Beard K. & Lee A., 2006). In contrast to ADRs that cause clinical presentations that require immediate emergency admission, such as Stevens-Johnson syndrome (Del Pozzo Magana, Lazo Langner, Carleton, Castro-Pastrana, & Rieder, 2011), and metabolic or neurological ADRs, which require close monitoring (Pringsheim, Doja, et al., 2011; Pringsheim, Panagiotopoulos, et al., 2011), the conceptualization that ADRs can significantly affect behavior has not yet been established in pediatrics. Interestingly, the terminology of behavioral ADRs was not used in any of the charts of the 17 analyzed patients, although this was the likely reason for the frequent medication changes and the high number of prescriptions. Instead, terminology such as "allergy," "intolerance," and "parent concern" was used when discussing impacts of medications. A 16-year-old patient from our cohort who was described as experiencing reduced amounts of sleep and also nonrestorative sleep ("falling asleep can take him from one to two hours") had a severe ADR to mixed amphetamine salts (Adderall XR®). This ADR encompassed twitches in his limbs and entire body and shivering and restlessness for hours, followed by emotional breakdown with uninterrupted sleep, and finally amnesia. Following this event, the patient was diagnosed by medical staff in the hospital with Tourette's syndrome and an "allergic reaction" to mixed amphetamine salts. He and his family were not counseled about the possibility of similar symptomatic episodes in the case of future use of psychostimulants. This case illustrates that even neurological ADRs that present clinically as fairly dramatic effects, such as akathisia (a feeling of internal restlessness) (Keller et al., 2013; Miller & Fleischhacker, 2000), are not established in pediatric and child psychiatry as ADRs.

The Challenge with the Accurate Diagnosis of a Sleep Problem and its Treatment. In current clinical practice, professional exploratory models are based on previously established clinical diagnoses and bias toward categorical daytime diagnoses. Integration of sleep and wake phenotypes in behavioral, neurological, and mental health assessments is not currently the standard of care. Screening tools for assessing sleep/wake behaviors in children were initially introduced a decade ago (Owens & Dalzell, 2005); however, systematic research to describe the clinical characteristics of sleep problems in children with neurodevelopmental conditions started very recently with the development of specific clinical tools for in-depth assessment of children and adolescents with neurodevelopmental conditions (Blankenburg et al., 2013; Galland, Meredith-Jones, Terrill, & Taylor, 2014; Ipsiroglu et al., 2012).

The case vignette demonstrates the problem effectively; sleep problems were existent since early toddlerhood in the narratives and typically mentioned later in the medical records, after diagnosing challenging/disruptive daytime behaviors, mainly ADHD, but also oppositional defiant and obsessive-compulsive disorders, was described to the family (but not formally diagnosed). At our clinic, to refine clinical assessment concepts (Ipsiroglu et al., 2013), we use qualitative methodology (therapeutic emplotment) and a home-based video recording system (videosomnography) to capture sleep behaviors and movement patterns. Therapeutic emplotment allows patients and caregivers to tell the story and explain their perspectives. This information is then transformed into a medical report, which is shared with the patient to check for correct understanding of his or her observations. In addition, videosomnography acts as an extended eye during the sleep situation, allowing us to record and analyze movement patterns, and has been instrumental in approaching and understanding the sequelae of WED (Galland et al., 2014). In summary, we are applying the clinical skills of listening, observing, exploring, and describing, as physicians have always done; however, today time constrictions make this practice fairly challenging.

CONCLUSION AND OUTLOOK

From our analysis of worst case scenarios we conclude: (1) desperate clinical circumstances often lead to deviations from common prescription recommendations, such as prescribing more than two psychostimulants at a time or starting with off-label prescription of antipsychotics to very young children; (2) the variety of pathophysiologies and etiologies causing sleep problems and the strong interdependence of sleep and wake behaviors require new assessment methodologies, targeted treatment strategies, and monitoring of treatment effects and adverse effects; and (3) monitoring of prescription and over- the-counter medication effectiveness and adverse effects, including the in sleep/

wake behaviors, is a way to overcome the current overmedication cycles and polypharmacy. Digital home-based technologies (apps) linked with clinical databases will facilitate the assessment of practice-related outcomes and act as a powerful tool for quality-of-care improvement, as the Cancer Foundation Registry and Cystic Fibrosis Foundation Registry have proven (Cystic Fibrosis Canada, 2011; Statistics Canada, 2012). A similar database for children with FASDs or other neurodevelopmental conditions who require medication may be a powerful vehicle in the establishment of functional sleep/wake behavior assessment screening before starting medications and support the implementation of evidence-based criteria for diagnosis and treatment of sleep-related daytime sequelae (DiPietro & Illes, 2014; Ho et al., 2011; Pringsheim, Doja, et al., 2011; Pringsheim, Panagiotopoulos, et al., 2011; updates to the CAMESA guidelines are available at www.camesaguideline.org).

REFERENCES

Aagaard, L., & Hansen, E. H. (2011). The occurrence of adverse drug reactions reported for attention deficit hyperactivity disorder (ADHD) medications in the pediatric population: A qualitative review of empirical studies. *Neuropsychiatric Disease and Treatment, 7*(1), 729–744.

Allen, R. P., Picchietti, D. L., Garcia-Borreguero, D., Ondo, W. G., Walters, A. S., Winkelman, J. W., et al. (2014). Restless legs syndrome/Willis-Ekbom disease diagnostic criteria: Updated International Restless Legs Syndrome Study Group (IRLSSG) consensus criteria—history, rationale, description, and significance. *Sleep Medicine, 15*(8), 860–873.

Allen, R. P., Walters, A. S., Montplaisir, J., Hening, W., Montplaisir, J., Hening, W., et al. (2005). Restless legs syndrome prevalence and impact: REST general population study. *Archives of Internal Medicine, 165*(11), 1286–1292.

American Academy of Sleep Medicine. (2005). International classification of sleep disorders. *Diagnostic and coding manual* (2nd ed.). Westchester, IL: American Academy of Sleep Medicine.

Beard, K., & Lee, A. (2006). In A. Lee (Ed.), *Adverse drug reactions*. London: Pharmaceutical Press.

Blankenburg, M., Tietze, A. L., Hechler, T., Hirschfeld, G., Michel, E., Koh, M., et al. (2013). Snake: The development and validation of a questionnaire on sleep disturbances in children with severe psychomotor impairment. *Sleep Medicine, 14*(4), 339–351.

Bruni, O., & Novelli, L. (2010). Sleep disorders in children. *Clinical Evidence (Online)*, 2010, 2304.

Brunt L. & Steger B. (Eds.). (2008). *Worlds of sleep*. Berlin, Germany: Timme GmbH.

Buscemi, N., & Witmans, M. (2006). What is the role of melatonin in the management of sleep disorders in children? *Paediatrics & Child Health, 11*(8), 517–519.

CADDRA, Canadian ADHD Resource Alliance, Canadian ADHD Practice Guidelines. (2011). http://www.caddra.ca/pdfs/caddraGuidelines2011.pdf.

Centers for Disease Control and Prevention. (2013). *Attention-deficit/hyperactivity disorder (ADHD): Recommendations from the American Academy of Pediatrics (AAP)*. Atlanta: Centers for Disease Control and Prevention.

Chen, M. L., Olson, H. C., Picciano, J. F., Starr, J. R., & Owens, J. (2012). Sleep problems in children with fetal alcohol spectrum disorders. *Journal of Clinical Sleep Medicine, 8*(4), 421–429.

Chudley, A., Conry, J., Cook, J., Loock, C., Rosales, T., & LeBlanc, N. (2005). Fetal alcohol spectrum disorder: Canadian guidelines for diagnosis. *CMAJ, 172*(5), S1–S21.

Clarren, S. K., & Smith, D. W. (1978). The fetal alcohol syndrome. *The Lamp*, *35*(10), 4–7.

Coles, C. D. (2001). Fetal alcohol exposure and attention: Moving beyond ADHD. *Alcohol Research & Health*, *25*(3), 199–203.

Cystic Fibrosis Canada. (2011). *The Canadian Cysic Fibrosis Registry: 2011 annual report.* Toronto: Cystic Fibrosis Canada. Retrieved from http://www.cysticfibrosis.ca/wpcontent/uploads/2013/10/Registry2011FINALOnlineEN.pdf.

Del Pozzo Magana, B. R., Lazo Langner, A., Carleton, B., Castro-Pastrana, L. I., & Rieder, M. J. (2011). A systematic review of treatment of drug-induced Stevens-Johnson syndrome and toxic epidermal necrolysis in children. *Journal of Population Therapeutics and Clinical Pharmacology*, *18*, e121–e133.

DiPietro, N., Illes, J., & for the Canadian Working Group on Antipsychotic Medications and Children. (2014). Rising antipsychotic prescriptions for children and youth: cross-sectoral solutions for a multimodal problem. *CMAJ*, *186*, 653–654; Epub ahead of print March 24, 2014.

Doig, J., McLennan, J. D., & Gibbard, W. B. (2008). Medication effects of symptoms of attention deficit/hyperactivity disorder in children with a fetal alcohol spectrum disorder. *Journal of Child and Adolescent Psychopharmacology*, *18*(4), 365–371.

Findling, R. L., Horwitz, S. M., Birmaher, B., Kowatch, R. A., Fristad, M. A., Youngstrom, E. A., et al. (2011). Clinical characteristics of children receiving antipsychotic medication. *Journal of Child and Adolescent Psychopharmacology*, *21*(4), 311–319.

Galland, B., Meredith-Jones, K., Terrill, P., & Taylor, R. (2014). Challenges and emerging technologies within the field of pediatric actigraphy. *Frontiers in Psychiatry*, *5*, 99.

Gringras, P., Gamble, C., Jones, A. P., Wiggs, L., Williamson, P. R., Sutcliffe, A., et al. (2012). Melatonin for sleep problems in children with neurodevelopmental disorders: Randomised double masked placebo controlled trial. *BMJ*, *345*, 6664.

Hellemans, K. G., Sliwowska, J. H., Verma, P., & Weinberg, J. (2010). Prenatal alcohol exposure: Fetal programming and later life vulnerability to stress, depression and anxiety disorders. *Neuroscience and Biobehavioral Reviews*, *34*(6), 791–807.

Hill, R. M., Hegemier, S., & Tennyson, L. M. (1989). The fetal alcohol syndrome: A multihandicapped child. *Neurotoxicology*, *10*(3), 585–595.

Ho, J., Panagiotopoulos, C., McCrindle, B., Grisaru, S., McCrindle, B., Grisaru, S., et al. (2011). Management recommendations for metabolic complications associated with second-generation antipsychotic use in children and youth. *Paediatrics & Child Health*, *16*(9), 575–580.

Ipsiroglu, O. S., Carey, N., Collet, J. P., Fast, D., Garden, J., Jan, J. E., et al. (2012). De-medicalizing sleep: Sleep assessment tools in the community setting for clients (patients) with FASD & prenatal substance exposure. *NOFAS-UK: Fetal alcohol forum*, 33–41.

Ipsiroglu, O. S., McKellin, W. H., Carey, N., & Loock, C. (2013). "They silently live in terror…" why sleep problems and night-time related quality-of-life are missed in children with a fetal alcohol spectrum disorder. *Social Science and Medicine*, *79*, 76–83.

Jan, J. E., Asante, K. O., Conry, J. L., Fast, D. K., Bax, M. C. O., Ipsiroglu, O. S., et al. (2010). Sleep health issues for children with FASD: Clinical considerations. *International Journal of Pediatrics*, *2010*, 1–7.

Jan, J. E., Bax, M. C., Owens, J. A., Ipsiroglu, O. S., & Wasdell, M. B. (2012). Neurophysiology of circadian rhythm sleep disorders of children with neurodevelopmental disabilities. *European Journal of Paediatric Neurology*, *16*(5), 403–412.

Jan, J. E., Owens, J. A., Weiss, M. D., Johnson, K. P., Wasdell, M. B., Freeman, R. D., et al. (2008). Sleep hygiene for children with neurodevelopmental disabilities. *Pediatrics*, *122*(6), 1343–1350.

Jones, K. L., & Smith, D. W. (1973). Recognition of the fetal alcohol syndrome in early infancy. *Lancet, 302*(7836), 999–10001.

Keller, D. M., Myhre, K. E., Dowben, J. S., Keltner, N. L., Myhre, K. E., Dowben, J. S., et al. (2013). Biological perspectives: Akathisia: Ants in your pants. *Perspectives in Psychiatric Care, 49*(3), 149–151.

LaFrance, M. A., McLachlan, K., Nash, K., Andrew, G., Loock, C., Oberlander, T. F., et al. (2014). Evaluation of the neurobehavioural screening tool in children with fetal alcohol spectrum disorders (FASD). *Journal of Population Therapeutics and Clinical Pharmacology, 20*(2), 197–210.

Magnus, L. (1999). Nonepileptic uses of gabapentin. *Epilepsia, 40*(Suppl. 6), S66–S72, discussion S73–S74.

May, P. A., Gossage, J. P., Kalberg, W. O., Robinson, L. K., Buckley, D., Manning, M., et al. (2009). Prevalence and epidemiologic characteristics of FASD from various research methods with an emphasis on recent in-school studies. *Developmental Disabilities Research Reviews, 15*(3), 176.

Michaud, M. (2006). Is the suggested immobilization test the "gold standard" to assess restless legs syndrome? *Sleep Medicine, 7*(7), 541–543.

Miller, C. H., & Fleischhacker, W. W. (2000). Managing antipsychotic-induced acute and chronic akathisia. *Drug Safety, 22*, 73–81.

O'Connor, M. J., & Paley, B. (2009). Psychiatric conditions associated with prenatal alcohol exposure. *Developmental Disabilities Research Reviews, 15*(3), 225–234.

Oldani, M. J. (2009). Uncanny scripts: Understanding pharmaceutical emplotment in the aboriginal context. *Transcultural Psychiatry, 46*(1), 131–156.

O'Malley, K. D. (1997). Safety of combined pharmacotherapy. *Journal of the American Academy of Child and Adolescent Psychiatry, 36*(11), 1489–1490.

O'Malley, K. D., Koplin, B., & Dohner, V. A. (2000). Psychostimulant clinical response in fetal alcohol syndrome. *Canadian Journal of Psychiatry, 45*(1), 90–91.

O'Malley, K. D., & Nanson, J. (2002). Clinical implications of a link between fetal alcohol spectrum disorder and attention-deficit hyperactivity disorder. *Canadian Journal of Psychiatry, 47*(4), 349–354.

O'Malley, K., Streissguth, A. (2003). Clinical intervention and support for children aged zero to five years with fetal alcohol spectrum disorder and their parents/caregivers. In Tremblay R. E., Barr R. G., & Peters R. (Eds.), *Encyclopedia on early childhood development [online]* (pp. 1–9). Montreal, Quebec: Centre of Excellence for Early Childhood Development. Available at: http://www.excellence-earlychildhood.ca/documents/Omalley-StreissguthANGxp.pdf.

Owens, J. A., & Dalzell, V. (2005). Use of 'BEARS' sleep screening tool in a pediatric resident' continuity clinic: A pilot study. *Sleep Medicine, 6*(1), 63–69.

Paley, B., & O'Connor, M. J. (2009). Intervention for individuals with fetal alcohol spectrum disorders: Treatment approaches and case management. *Developmental Disabilities Research Reviews, 15*, 258–267.

Picchietti, D. L. (2013). Restless legs syndrome and periodic limb movement disorder in children. In UpToDate, R. D. Chervin, & A. G. Hoppin (Eds.). Waltham, MA: UpToDate.

Picchietti, D. L., Allen, R. P., Walters, A. S., Davidson, J. E., Myers, A., & Ferini-Strambi, L. (2007). Restless legs syndrome: Prevalence and impact in children and adolescents—The Peds REST study. *Pediatrics, 120*, 253–266.

Picchietti, D. L., Arbuckle, R. A., Abetz, L., Durmer, J. S., Ivanenko, A., Owens, J. A., et al. (2011). Pediatric restless legs syndrome: Analysis of symptom descriptions and drawings. *Journal of Child Neurology, 26*(11), 1365–1376.

Picchietti, D. L., Bruni, O., de Weerd, A., Durmer, J. S., Kotagal, S., Durmer, J. S., et al. (2013). Pediatric restless legs syndrome diagnostic criteria: An update by the International Restless Legs Syndrome Study Group. *Sleep Medicine, 14*(12), 1253–1259.

Pringsheim, T., Doja, A., Belanger, S., Patten, S., & Canadian Alliance for Monitoring Effectiveness and Safety of Antipsychotics in Children (CAMESA) guideline group. (2011). Treatment recommendations for extrapyramidal side effects associated with second-generation antipsychotic use in children and youth. *Paediatrics & Child Health, 16*(9), 590–598.

Pringsheim, T., Panagiotopoulos, C., Davidson, J., Ho, J., & Canadian Alliance for Monitoring Effectiveness and Safety of Antipsychotics in Children (CAMESA) guideline group. (2011). Evidence-based recommendations for monitoring safety of second-generation antipsychotics in children and youth. *Paediatrics & Child Health, 16*(9), 581–589.

Public Health Agency of Canada. (2005). Knowledge and attitudes of health professionals about fetal alcohol syndrome: Results of a national survey. *Fetal alcohol spectrum disorder (FASD).* Ottawa, Ontario: Health Canada.

Rasmussen, C., Andrew, G., Zwaigenbaum, L., & Tough, S. (2008). Neurobehavioral outcomes of children with fetal alcohol spectrum disorders: A Canadian perspective. *Journal of Paediatrics and Child Health, 13*(3), 185–191.

Rasmussen, C., Benz, J., Pei, J., Andrew, G., Schuller, G., Abele-Webster, L., et al. (2010). The impact of an ADHD co-morbidity on the diagnosis of FASD. *The Canadian Journal of Clinical Pharmacology, 17*(1), 165–176.

Robinson, A. A., & Malow, B. A. (2012). Gabapentin shows promise in treating refractory insomnia in children. *Journal of Child Neurology, 28*(12), 1618–1621.

Ronsley, R., Scott, D., Warburton, W. P., Hamdi, R. D., Louie, D. C., Davidson, J., et al. (2013). A population-based study of antipsychotic prescription trends in children and adolescents in British Columbia, from 1996 to 2011. *Canadian Journal of Psychiatry, 58*(6), 361–369.

Rowles, B. M., & Findling, R. L. (2010). Review of pharmacotherapy options for the treatment of attention-deficit/hyperactivity disorder (ADHD) and ADHD-like symptoms in children and adolescents with developmental disorders. *Developmental Disabilities Research Reviews, 16,* 273–282.

Ryan, S., & Ferguson, D. L. (2006). The person behind the face of fetal alcohol spectrum disorder: Student experiences and family and professionals' perspectives on FASD. *Rural Special Education Quarterly, 25*(1), 32.

Statistics Canada. (2012). *Canadian Cancer Registry (CCR): Detailed information for 2010.* Ottawa: Health Statistics Division, Statistics Canada. Retrieved from http://www23.statcan.gc.ca:81/imdb/p2SV.pl?Function=getSurvey&SDDS=3207&lang=en&db=imdb&adm=8&dis=2.

Steinhausen, H. C., & Spohr, H. L. (1998). Long-term outcome of children with fetal alcohol syndrome: Psychopathology, behavior, and intelligence. *Alcoholism: Clinical and Experimental Research, 22*(2), 334–338.

Streissguth, A. P., Barr, H. M., Kogan, J., & Bookstein, F. L. (1996). *Understanding the occurrence of secondary disabilities in clients with fetal alcohol syndrome (FAS) and fetal alcohol effects (FAE): Final report.* Seattle, WA: University of Washington Publication Services.

Subcommittee on Attention-Deficit/Hyperactivity Disorder; Steering Committee on Quality Improvement and Management, Wolraich, M., Brown, L., Brown, R.T., Dupaul, G., Earls, M., et al. (2011). ADHD: Clinical practice guideline for the diagnosis, evaluation, and treatment of attention-deficit/hyperactivity disorder in children and adolescents. *Pediatrics, 128*(5), 1007–1022.

Therapeutics Initiative. (2009). Increasing use of newer antipsychotics in children: A cause for concern? Therapeutics Letter #74.

Tilma, J., Tilma, K., Norregaard, O., & Ostergaard, J. R. (2013). Early childhood-onset restless legs syndrome: Symptoms and effect of oral iron treatment. *Acta Paediatrica, 102,* 221–226.

Parents/caregivers. In R. E. Tremblay, R. G. Barr, R. De., & V. Peters (Eds.), *Encyclopedia on early childhood development* (rev ed.) (pp. 1–9). Montreal, Quebec: Centre of Excellence for Early Childhood Development (online).

Walters, A. S., Silvestri, R., Zucconi, M., Chandrashekariah, R., Konofal, E., Silvestri, R., et al. (2008). Review of the possible relationship and hypothetical links between attention deficit hyperactivity disorder (ADHD) and the simple sleep related movement disorders, parasomnias, hypersomnias, and circadian rhythm disorders. *Journal of Clinical Sleep Medicine*, *4*(6), 591–600.

Wengel, T., Hanlon-Dearman, A. C., & Fjelsted, B. (2011). Sleep and sensory characteristics in young children with fetal alcohol spectrum disorder. *Journal of Developmental and Behavioral Pediatrics*, *32*(5), 384–392.

Wiggs, L. (2001). Sleep problems in children with developmental disorders. *Journal of the Royal Society of Medicine*, *94*(4), 177–179.

Wiggs, L., & Stores, G. (1996). Severe sleep disturbance and daytime challenging behavior in children with severe learning disabilities. *Journal of Intellectual Disability Research*, *40*(6), 518–528.

Wilens, T. E., Spencer, T., Biederman, J., Wozniak, J., & Connor, D. (1995). Combined pharmacotherapy: An emerging trend in pediatric psychopharmacology. *Journal of the American Academy of Child and Adolescent Psychiatry*, *34*(1), 110–112.

Zhang, T., Smith, M. A., Camp, P. G., Shajari, S., MacLeod, S. M., & Carleton, B. C. (2013). Prescription drug dispensing profiles for one million children: A population-based analysis. *European Journal of Clinical Pharmacology*, *69*(3), 581–588.

Zucconi, M., & Bruni, O. (2001). Sleep disorders in children with neurologic diseases. *Seminars in Pediatric Neurology*, *8*(4), 258–275.

Chapter 7

Implementing Change in Prescribing Practices

Andrea Murphy[*,†], **David Gardner**[*,†], **Stan Kutcher**[†,‡,¶]

[*]College of Pharmacy, Department of Psychiatry, Dalhousie University, Halifax, Nova Scotia, Canada
[†]Department of Psychiatry, Dalhousie University, Halifax, Nova Scotia, Canada
[‡]Sun Life Chair in Adolescent Mental Health, IWK Health Centre and Dalhousie University, Halifax, Nova Scotia, Canada
[¶]WHO Collaborating Center, IWK Health Centre—Maritime Outpatient Psychiatry, Halifax, Nova Scotia, Canada

INTRODUCTION

Psychotropic medicines such as antipsychotics are essential components of the management plan for many people with mental illness, for managing symptoms, supporting recovery, and maintaining wellness. As with any intervention in health care, there are uncertainties for each individual user related to the benefits and risks associated with their use. In this book, concerns are raised about the marked increase in the use of antipsychotics for an expanding collection of nonpsychotic indications in children and youth, with questions of effectiveness, safety, and place in therapy. These trends are worrisome and challenge us to re-examine how these medications should be used. Implicit in this challenge are the following questions: (1) how effective are antipsychotics in youth of different ages with different clinical presentations?; (2) what is their place in therapy relative to alternative management approaches?; (3) what are best practices in treatment selection, initiation, maintenance, and discontinuation?; and (4) how do we translate and widely implement the answers to the preceding questions in clinical practice? It is this last challenge regarding implementing changes in clinical practice related to the use of antipsychotics in children and adolescents that we focus on in this chapter, by providing strategies and frameworks to use when attempting to create change.

Changing any part of the health system toward achieving best practice supported by an evidence-informed approach is complex, whether we anticipate, recognize, or inherit problems within the system. Making changes in the way we use medicines in the broader health system is inherently complex because of the

The Science and Ethics of Antipsychotic Use in Children. http://dx.doi.org/10.1016/B978-0-12-800016-8.00007-6
149

multiple factors influencing their use, many of which we do not yet adequately understand (such as the preferences and priorities of youth and families); we are therefore less able to determine what should be a part of "best practice." A pragmatic approach toward rational use of medicines, including antipsychotics, and standard principles of prescribing includes use of the best available evidence for efficacy and safety, implementation of a systematic monitoring scheme at the patient level, and a sophisticated surveillance system at the population level to track treatment outcomes and adverse events. These approaches, while necessary and encouraged, are challenged by the relatively limited amount of high-quality research involving children and youth and their unique social and developmental considerations related to the contexts in which these medicines are used.

The path to improving the use of antipsychotic medication in the treatment of young people is thus much more complicated than simply delivering an educational program targeting prescribers and expecting best practice care as a result. In this chapter, we explore the phenomenon of changing prescriber behavior and use the prescribing of antipsychotics in young people to exemplify a stepwise approach to behavior change, with a focus on individuals in the broader health care context. However, we must remain cognizant that changing prescribing behavior is only one piece of a comprehensive system-wide change affecting sociocultural, technical, economic, political, and legal interests and influences that must occur to realize overall improvements in the mental health care and outcomes of young people and families living with mental illness (Kutcher & McLuckie, 2010, 2011).

PHARMACOTHERAPEUTIC DECISION MAKING

Before attempting to address issues related to prescribing practices and work toward changing prescribing behavior, it is important to understand the phenomenon of "prescribing" and psychotropic use decision making, including the circumstances in which it occurs and the factors that influence that process. The opportunity for psychopharmacological prescribing occurs after the youth and/ or the parent/caregiver "enters the system." Through a simplistic representation, Figure 7.1 shows typical mechanisms in the Canadian healthcare system by which a patient may engage with the system, including potential referrals or transitions within and among providers in the system. Inherently, there is high variability in terms of the availability, realized access, and equitable distribution of these services throughout Canada. The time needed to access service is also highly variable within and among provinces and territories in Canada.

The opportunity to prescribe antipsychotics occurs as part of the assessment and treatment plan, which ideally is developed and delivered under the direction of a psychiatric specialist or a prescriber who has the requisite capability and competency. This goes beyond prescribing the right medicine at the right time, dose, and duration. Prescribers must take into account numerous other factors, including but not limited to availability of psychiatric specialty providers and

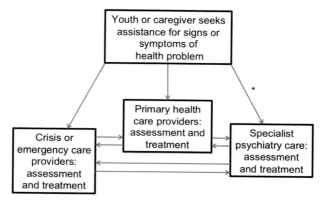

FIGURE 7.1   Youth presentation to the health care system. (*Specialist psychiatry care services are typically only easily accessible to those previously, and usually recently, receiving those services. This figure does not provide a visual representation for wait times affiliated with these services, which can be variable in length.)

treatment alternatives, effectiveness and safety data, patient and family treatment preferences, and financial implications. Addressing shortcomings in system structures and processes frequently makes meeting the health needs and care preferences of youth and families very difficult, if not impossible. Thus, we rely on existing published research to help us better understand how prescribers and young people and their families engage in decision making about the use of medications, and to better understand current practice and ways to improve it.

Several widely accepted albeit general models and frameworks exist for understanding pharmacotherapeutic medicine use and decision making in clinical encounters, such as the authority/pharmacotherapy care model. These models and frameworks provide insights regarding the various stages in the treatment process and factors that influence these stages and treatment decisions (Einarson, 2005; Metge & Sketris, 2007; Sketris, Langille Ingram, Lummis, & Health Council of Canada, 2007; Sketris, Langille Ingram, & Lummis, 2009). For psychotropic medicines, several groups have attempted to explicate important influences and processes in decision making of patients through examining the patient experience. Relevant examples to this chapter include the experiences of adults taking antidepressants (Malpass et al., 2009) in which decisional steps including seeking help, accepting treatment, continuing treatment, and deciding to stop are defined, and the experiences of adolescents treated with psychotropic medications in which there is a sociocultural, personal, and interpersonal matrix of adolescent medication management and experience is described (Floersch et al., 2009). What is often not explicit within this literature is an understanding or description of the "patient-physician relationship" and the manner in which prescribers and patients interact to make decisions, or even the impact of involved caretakers, such as parents, on those interactions. We default to an existent way of conceptualizing decision making by one of three models:

(1) traditional (or paternalistic), (2) shared decision making, or (3) relatively informed choice[1] (Charles, Gafni, & Whelan, 1999).

In each of these models, the roles of the patient (and/or parents or caregivers) and the prescriber differ. In the traditional medical model, the role of the prescriber is active but the patient is passive, and the responsibility for the decision to medicate lies with the prescriber (Hamann, Leucht, & Kissling, 2003). In the shared and relatively informed decision-making models, however, patients and families have an active role in determining if and which medication is right for them. In these contexts, prescribers either play an active role in the shared decision-making approach or a more passive one in the relatively informed choice method. Decision responsibility lies primarily with the patient or family in the relatively informed choice method but is shared to a greater extent with the prescriber with the shared decision-making approach.

There is variability in the application of various decision-making approaches in psychiatric care (Hamann et al., 2003). In the schizophrenia literature, shared and paternalistic (or traditional) decision-making models are often the preferred approaches and use of medicines is primarily directed by patient characteristics and not by patient choice (Hamann et al., 2009, 2012). However, this has been examined primarily in adult patients and has not, to our knowledge, been reported in studies of young people and their families, or for conditions other than schizophrenia in which antipsychotic medications are indicated. Based on our knowledge, there has yet to be substantial research on the application of shared decision-making models to children who are being treated with psychotropics (Moses, 2011) or on the topic of antipsychotic treatment and decision making involving young people and their families.

Decision making regarding the use of antipsychotics for children and youth is complicated by patient age, the nature and severity of illness, capacity to understand the illness and treatment options, health literacy and numeracy, involvement of parents and other family members, legal issues, preconceptions of treatment effectiveness and safety, understanding and conceptualization of symptoms, how youth make meaning of their illness experience and what meaning they get out of taking medications, and stigma, including self-stigma. Existing models and frameworks of treatment decision making do not adequately address these issues. Figure 7.2 outlines some additional, albeit not exhaustive, factors influencing prescribing decisions that in our collective experience and reading of available child- and youth-focused research are relevant to antipsychotic prescribing in this population. Some factors overlap and some are dependent on one another. Some may play out differently in different situations. For example, kinetic, dynamic, and genomic properties relating to medicines may be assessed from scientific studies but, once prescribed to an

---

[1] We have chosen to modify the phrase "informed choice" to "relatively informed choice" as it is effectively impossible for young people and their families to have a fully informed choice given the complexities and sheer volume of information involved.

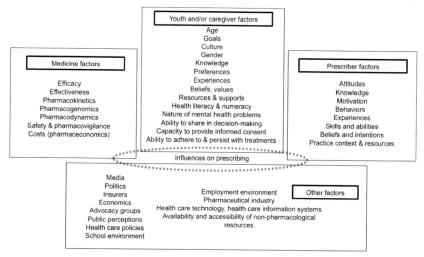

FIGURE 7.2   Potential factors influencing antipsychotic prescribing to children and adolescents.

individual, can have different results from those obtained in laboratory or controlled trial conditions. Similarly, an individualist approach to an adolescent that is based on Western cultural norms may not be as acceptable to parents from other sociocultural groups that emphasize a collectivist, parent-driven approach. It is also important to recognize the dynamic nature of these factors; they do not remain static and evolve over time as new information, evidence, and changes in social and economic influences can alter their impact or level of influence in the decision-making process. Only more recently have youth and/or caregiver experiences and physician experiences with these medicines been explored in scholarship.

THE YOUTH AND FAMILY EXPERIENCE OF PSYCHOTROPIC DECISION MAKING

The role of the child or youth in psychotropic-related decision making is an under-researched area. Similar to adults, youth experience various decision points (i.e., seeking help, accepting, continuing, and stopping treatment) during which they make pharmacotherapeutic management decisions, both overtly and covertly, and negotiate the world of medical intervention, seen through a lens of self-awareness that has been called the "medicated self" (Malpass et al., 2009). This self-awareness is in itself a complex phenomenon, influenced by factors as diverse as personality, belief systems, and the social ecology in which the young person exists. Some of these factors have been suggested as important to either not starting psychotropic medications or to deviations from the suggested treatment plan, including discontinuation of potentially effective interventions. These have been identified as including but not limited to perceived need for the medication, perceived helpfulness of the medication, desire for receiving a medication, desire for alleviation of disease experience, availability of choice in decision making pertaining to taking a medication, stigma related to the illness and to the treatment of the illness, mistrust of prescribers, and mistrust of makers or purveyors of medicines (separate from concerns about adverse effects) (Longhofer & Floersch, 2010; Moses, 2011).

In addition to acknowledging youth-specific factors influencing the use of psychotropics in this population, we must take into account how parents or caregivers influence this decision-making process. Indeed, parent/caretaker influences work through and interact with many of the factors previously identified and the outcome of the decision is the result of the complex interplay among these many factors. Parent/caretaker influences in the decision-making process may be similar or in direct contrast to factors motivating youth toward certain decisions. In our research, we explored the lived experience of taking antipsychotic medicines through a series of interviews with youth and parents. Their responses indicated that youth were not adequately informed or consulted regarding antipsychotic therapy decisions. They described persisting and frustrating gaps in their knowledge about the potential benefits and harms of the various medication treatment options, thereby limiting their ability to make well-informed, self-determined decisions. In part, this may account for the expressed ambivalence by youth, and also by parents, regarding treatment decisions that involve initiating, continuing, changing, and stopping medications (Murphy et al., 2015).

In our research, both youth and parents expressed concerns regarding difficulties accessing and remaining connected to specialty care. Multiple issues were voiced about the capacity, interest, and capabilities of primary care providers in providing safe and effective mental health care to youth with serious mental illnesses. Some of those interviewed reported "manipulating" the system to ensure that young persons who were doing well symptomatically and functionally stayed connected to specialty care for as long as possible to avoid being wait-listed if and when symptoms and functioning deteriorated. In part, this well-recognized delay in accessing specialty mental health services may be due to a lack of primary healthcare capacity in the diagnosis and treatment of common non-serious mental disorders, thus leaving young people and families with no place to turn but to specialty services. This high-volume crush of lower-intensity specialty care in turn limits access to appropriate services for young people and families experiencing severe or complex mental disorders (Kutcher, 2011).

Taken as a whole, our combined extensive clinical experience and qualitative research highlight the need for understanding how to more effectively involve youth and parent participation in decision making related to treatment with psychotropic medications, including antipsychotics. Our data and experience indicate the need for improved communications that support a better understanding of and response to patient and parent/caregiver needs, concerns, and expectations. Better communications will support more efficient and effective self-management and use of the healthcare system throughout treatment.

Unfortunately, there exist almost no data from appropriately designed research that can help us better understand what effect an empowered and engaged youth and/or family can have on the prescriber's approach to therapeutic decision making. We also have little or no information on the prescriber or health system dimensions of this interaction. Far more work is needed examining the experiences of youth prescribed psychotropic medications and the experiences of their families and their prescribers to help us better understand these issues.

The school environment is another important factor that can impact the use of and attitudes toward medications for mental illness (antipsychotics or otherwise) in youth. While school policies may forbid teaching personnel and other school staff from making health recommendations directly, indirect methods can instigate student mental health assessment and parental support for the initiation of psychotropic medications. Off-handed comments from teachers or others, such as "did you forget your meds today?" or "do you need to up your dose?," have a substantial impact on the student's self-esteem and sense of self and safety and may contribute to treatment refusal. Other school and medication-related issues include but are not limited to policies about the administration of medications at school, stigma related to both the understanding of mental disorders and the use of medications in their treatments, and generally low levels of mental health literacy in both students and teachers (Wei, Kutcher, & Szumilas, 2011). Recent research reports, however, have demonstrated that some of these issues may be positively and sustainably addressed by applying a mental health literacy curriculum intervention in junior high and secondary schools (Kutcher & Wei, 2014). Further school-related interventions, such as seminars for teachers about psychotropic medications during educator mental health conferences, have shown promising results, as have programs embedding mental health competencies in identification, triage, referral, and support of youth with mental illnesses (Kutcher, Wei, & Weist, in press). See Appendix A for a link to access curriculum resources.

In our qualitative research to date, several youth have also discussed the influence of employment on their medication-taking experiences and decisions. As for school, antipsychotic medications can support the ability to function well at work but can also impair occupational functioning. The decision to disclose mental health information, including diagnosis or medications by class or name, is a recurrent and understandably anxiety-provoking concern for young people that may lead to job insecurity or medication non-adherence. Further work is needed to determine the impact of the workplace on youth with mental illness, as this area is largely unexplored (Canadian Standards Association, 2013).

THE PRESCRIBER EXPERIENCE OF PSYCHOTROPICS AND DECISION MAKING

Prescriber comfort and experience with the use of antipsychotics in children and youth is important to understand and can be highly variable, given the range of training, clinical experiences, and ongoing professional development activities as well as individual factors that are involved. Many prescriptions for psychotropic medications, including antipsychotics, are initiated and/or continued by non-psychiatric specialists, particularly general practitioners. In our data from psychiatrists and general practitioners regarding their experiences of prescribing antipsychotics to youth, we found that psychotropics, despite concerns over the potential for more harm than benefit, are often used due to the lack of access to non-pharmacological services and resources. Moreover, our research indicates that many physicians take youth preferences into consideration when making decisions about treatment. However, what remains unclear is the extent to which these preferences are obtained consistently and systematically and under what conditions they influence treatment decisions. Are they obtained prior to discussions about treatment alternatives or do physicians seek to align preferences and risk avoidance following a discussion of potential risks and benefits? Physician preferences and previous patient experiences contribute significantly to the discussion of therapeutic alternatives and the development of personal formularies that reconcile or determine advantages and disadvantages of therapies, which can occur before presenting treatment alternatives to patients and/ or their families. In one of our studies, a physician indicated, "I will admit to a couple of biases. I don't like risperidone," and went on to explain the experience of managing patients with galactorrhea, menstrual irregularities, erectile dysfunction, etc. Later, this physician also reported advantages of risperidone, "…I had a couple of people who are just on the cusp of exams, and we've gone to risperidone first line because they are less sedated on it than some others, and because your titration is quick." Another physician similarly discussed how experiences had influenced preferences: "I tend to stay away from olanzapine because I've had experience and… Well, I tend to use quetiapine. That is such a crap shoot. And I don't know… This is more like the art or the cookery, the recipe of medicine but I've had experience with clients becoming diabetic on olanzapine. And the weight gain is a big problem, and the carbohydrate craving and all of that. Risperidone, that caused a prolactin over-drive in a patient I worked with a few years ago, which was really troublesome to her. You know, her breasts started leaking milk. I think people who are struggling with some mind demons, having these physical experiences can make it really hard to sell the idea of a medication. I haven't tried Abilify—aripiprazole. I think that is the newest or one of the newer APs [antipsychotics]. I've not had experience with it." The statement "That is such a crap shoot. And I don't know… This is more like the art or the cookery…." also demonstrates the weighing of non-ideal choices and limited evidence for safety and effectiveness.

Family preferences were also discussed as influencing treatment selection, but this was considered on a case-by-case basis and dependent on the capabilities and capacity of the youth to make treatment decisions. There are also complexities of privacy and confidentiality when physicians are treating youth and their family members concurrently, especially in remote and rural areas. For example, a prescriber in our focus group from a rural area indicated, "And so often, the mom will come in without him and say what is going on… Like I kind of know what is going on a lot more than the kid knows I know because I have the mom coming in for her pap, and she's telling me, 'Guess what happened last week? He's doing this and this.'"

Similar to other literature in this area, the majority of decision making reported by physicians in our research appears to follow either the traditional decision-making model or the shared-decision approach. Much more research into prescriber factors and how various elements in the contexts of their practice influences them is necessary to help us develop a better understanding of this component of prescribing. Such studies should be of sufficient design quality to allow for analysis of all these factors and the potential interactions among them.

AN APPROACH TO DESIGNING STRATEGIES FOR CHANGING PRESCRIBING BEHAVIORS

Achieving positive behavior change in healthcare systems that involve patients, families, and clinicians is challenging. Before implementing interventions, which are often complex in nature and at times expensive, systematically classifying behaviors of interest and the contexts in which they occur provides useful insights into variables that influence the change process and lead to a desired outcome. For example, prior to attempting to make changes in prescribing patterns in a practice, it is important to know and understand what patterns and trends in prescribing behaviors occur, for what kinds of patients and in what circumstances, and the characteristics of the individuals doing the prescribing. It is also important to consider the characteristics of the practice environment in which the prescribers work and the characteristics of the outer healthcare context aimed at supporting patients who are potentially in need of antipsychotics. Behavior change frameworks can be used to identify factors that may limit or interfere with desired behavior changes. We have attempted to create such a process that draws on previously described theories and frameworks from a variety of research domains, which may be able to assist us in better understanding the issues related to prescription of antipsychotics for young people (Figure 7.3) (Abraham & Michie, 2008; Cane, O'Connor, & Michie, 2012; Craig et al., 2008; Damschroder et al., 2009; Michie, Ashford, et al., 2011; Michie, van Stralen, & West, 2011; Michie, Fixsen, Grimshaw, & Eccles, 2009; Michie et al., 2013).

The application of some existing theories and frameworks for organizational change may be able to provide useful information regarding factors that will potentially impact change in psychotropic prescribing. We have considered numerous approaches to attempt to develop a heuristic approach to better understanding of this issue. We are aware that our framework choices may reflect our biases and that we may not have considered some that may prove useful. However, we are comfortable that we have chosen a number of different frameworks that support our understanding of behavior change and its challenges. Others may choose differently and future considerations may be based on those choices.

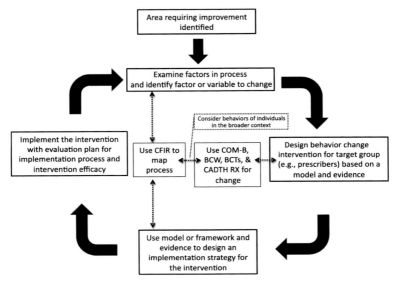

FIGURE 7.3   An approach to considering interventions for behavior change. COM-B: capability, opportunity, motivation–behavior; BCW: Behaviour Change Wheel; BCTs: behavior change techniques; CADTH Rx: Canadian Agency for Drugs and Technologies in Health Rx for Change database; CFIR: Consolidated Framework for Implementation Research.

Here, we outline frameworks that we consider useful for assisting in understanding the major system and individual factors that can impact prescribing behaviors. The Consolidated Framework for Implementation Research (CFIR) aims to translate the outcomes of health research into meaningful patient care across multiple settings and provides a foundation for understanding implementation (Damschroder et al., 2009). The framework emphasizes five key factors to consider for implementation: (1) the characteristics of interventions, (2) characteristics of individuals involved, (3) the inner setting (including structural and cultural factors), (4) the outer setting (including patient needs and resources, external policy, and incentives), and (5) the process by which implementation is accomplished (such as planning, engaging, and executing) (Figure 7.4) (Damschroder et al., 2009). The CFIR is directly relevant to implementing strategies aimed at improving prescribing. For example, the implementation of a guideline for the safe and effective use of antipsychotics in children and adolescents in community-based primary care practices would require specific knowledge and understanding of many environment, social, and other nonclinical factors. It is not sufficient or acceptable to presume uptake and use of a guideline, or any piece of research for that matter, just because it exists. Some of the key factors to consider for implementation are presented here and structured using the five key domains of the CFIR.

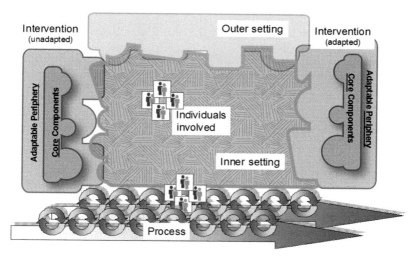

FIGURE 7.4 The consolidated framework for implementation research. From Damschroder et al. (2009), BioMed Central, Implementation Science.

With the guidelines as the intervention, we need to consider its characteristics, such as the evidence strength and quality within the guidelines and how they were developed, the relative advantage of the guidelines versus current practice in primary care clinics, and the adaptability of guideline recommendations to a specific clinical setting. Within the inner setting or the primary clinic environment, it is important to understand the characteristics of the practices, the culture, the networks and communications, the relative priority and perceived importance of implementing the guidelines by the clinic staff, and the degree to which practitioners perceive there is a need to change. The outer setting, which may include factors beyond the control of individual primary care practices, includes an assessment of the needs of and resources for patients, such as access and availability to other mental health services that the guidelines will undoubtedly include or make reference to, the extent to which practices are networked and linked with other external organizations within and outside of the formal mental healthcare system and are supported by these, and the potential pressures that push for guideline implementation such as those from professional organizations (e.g., APA's Choosing Wisely campaign; American Psychiatric Association, 2014). It is also critical to assess and understand the characteristics of individuals who will be implementing and using the guidelines. This includes but is not limited to beliefs and knowledge surrounding the guidelines, belief in personal capabilities for implementing and using guidelines, and personal readiness for change and use of the guidelines (from novice with little to no application of elements of the guideline, to expert with application of guidelines in a sustained fashion). It quickly becomes apparent after conducting an exercise such as this, using frameworks like the CFIR, that one may provide a structure for implementation that may extend into planning for evaluation of implementation (Damschroder et al., 2009).

Using this approach helps guide thinking about how to identify various factors that influence prescribing of antipsychotics to youth. Prescribers of psychotropic medications in Canada include general practitioners and specialists (including pediatricians and psychiatrists), as well as nurse practitioners. In some provinces other disciplines (e.g., pharmacists) have the ability to extend prescriptions so as to ensure continuity of care. These individual groups each receive a different quantity and quality of education, training, and mentoring in the use of antipsychotics pre- and post-licensure. Generally, they also experience different socialization within their own discipline and those experiences that occur in an interdisciplinary context. All of these factors as well as personal beliefs and values can contribute to prescribing of medications, including antipsychotics. These clinicians care for patients and families with a host of diagnoses in various health care settings that are influenced by organizational (e.g., health authority) policies alongside external influences from community organizations and broader social policies that impact community mental health (e.g., social services, schools, early childhood development programs). When we attempt to change prescribing behaviors, we must consider the design of interventions and that the likelihood for adoption depends on adaptability of the intervention to many of these contexts.

As with the guideline example of implementation above, all primary care clinics are not the same and, in keeping with CFIR terminology, will differ according to the individuals involved and the nature of the inner and outer settings. As we identify the range of contexts, we need to be able to determine the individual and collective impacts on prescribing behaviors. Here, the work of Michie and colleagues (2011) provides a comprehensive four-step approach to better understanding how prescribing behaviors may be modified (Table 7.1, Figure 7.5) in various contexts. This structured approach may be used to inform the design of interventions tasked with changing specific behaviors of prescribers.

In the first step we ask who needs to do what differently, when, where, and how. At first glance, it seems to be a simple exercise; however, as demonstrated by the CFIR example of guideline implementation, this needs to be carefully considered, planned, and implemented. As noted earlier, the range of prescribers for antipsychotics is variable, and prescribing activities that include initiating, continuing, and stopping antipsychotics may occur in a range of settings. Answering these questions requires the help of those working directly in the environments in which the prescribing occurs.

Within this stepwise approach by Michie and colleagues (2011), application of the "capability, opportunity, motivation—behavior" (COM-B) (Step 2, Table 7.1) allows us to develop an understanding of the prescribing behavior of individuals. The attempt is to understand why one does what one does and what needs to change for things to be done differently. In the COM-B, the capability

TABLE 7.1 Steps for Designing Interventions to Change Behavior

Steps	Activities
Step 1: Identify the target behaviors	Answer the questions: Who needs to do what differently? When, where, and how?
Step 2: Understand the target behaviors in context	Answer the questions: Why do we do what we do?
	What needs to change to do things differently?
	Conduct a COM-B assessment (Figure 7.5)
Step 3: Consider the full range of intervention functions	Use the Behaviour Change Wheel (Figure 7.6)
Step 4: Identify specific behavior change techniques	Use behavior change techniques

Michie, Ashford, et al., 2011; Michie, van Stralen, et al., 2011

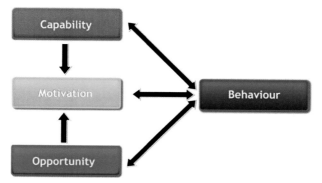

FIGURE 7.5   The COM-B system: a framework for understanding behavior. From Michie, van Stralen, et al. (2011), BioMed Central, Implementation Science.

(i.e., psychological or physical ability) to enact behaviors, the motivation (i.e., reflective and automatic mechanisms) that activates or inhibits a behavior, and the opportunity (i.e., physical and social environment) that enables a behavior are all be considered necessary components for a behavior to occur. Below we exemplify a COM-B assessment of antipsychotic prescribing to youth.

Capability assessment: Do prescribers know how to appropriately manage conditions in which antipsychotics may be indicated? Do they know how to appropriately prescribe antipsychotics and monitor patients taking antipsychotics? Do they know how to differentiate potential risks and benefits for a particular patient for a particular medicine? Are they capable of effectively informing youth and the family for the purpose of supporting shared treatment decisions?

Opportunity assessment: Do prescribers have access to resources to support appropriate management of conditions, including non-pharmacological management? Do prescribers have access to desirable medication options? Do prescribers have access to ongoing educational activities that include training in the optimal use of these medications?

Motivation assessment (examination of the beliefs, intentions, plans, wants, and needs of prescribers): How do prescribers decide when and how and for what conditions to use antipsychotics? Do prescribers believe these medicines will be helpful for their patients? Do prescribers believe that these medications are likely to be effective and safe for the patient in the condition prescribed? Do prescribers believe that non-pharmacological interventions are effective? What is the prescriber's reason for choosing to use a particular medication? What are the incentives and disincentives to this use? What are the habits of prescribers with regard to the use of antipsychotics in youth?

Following the COM-B assessment, we move on to consider a range of activities specifically designed to create interventions effective for achieving improved prescribing of antipsychotics to children and youth (Step 3, Table 7.1). To assist in this activity we refer to the Behaviour Change Wheel (BCW) developed by Michie and colleagues (2011), which identifies nine intervention functions to be considered (Figure 7.6). The use of this graphic may be associated

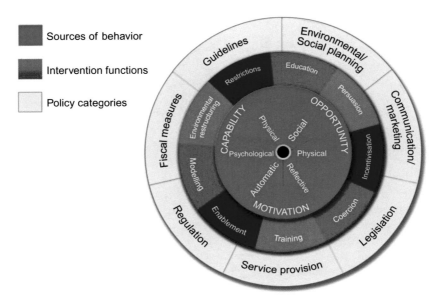

FIGURE 7.6   The Behaviour Change Wheel. From Michie, van Stralen, et al. (2011), BioMed Central, Implementation Science.

with application of a systematic approach to behavior change intervention design and implementation (Hendriks et al., 2013; Michie, Ashford, et al., 2011; Michie, van Stralen, et al., 2011).

The BCW has three concentric circles. The inner circle identifies factors intrinsically linked to behavior, the COM-B factors. The outer circle organizes policies that may influence behavior into a distinct set of familiar categories. In the middle circle are the intervention functions that may enable or support behavior change. We provide examples of how to use this graphic with consideration of both the COM-B assessment and intervention functions related to antipsychotic prescribing (Table 7.2).

TABLE 7.2 Intervention Functions with Potential Examples Related to Antipsychotic Prescribing

Intervention	Potential Model of Behavior Addressed (Michie, Ashford, et al., 2011; Michie, van Stralen, et al., 2011)	Examples of Potential Strategies Related to Antipsychotic Prescribing
Education	Psychological ability—capability Reflective—motivation	Continuing education session on antipsychotic medicines
Training	Psychological ability—capability Physical ability—capability	Workshop facilitated by experts with case-based learning on antipsychotic prescribing
Persuasion	Reflective—motivation Automatic—motivation	Send prescribers literature with graphs regarding adverse events (e.g., weight gain) of antipsychotics
Incentivization	Reflective—motivation Automatic—motivation	Use pay for performance incentives to achieve patient monitoring targets with antipsychotics prescribing
Coercion	Reflective—motivation Automatic—motivation	Retraction or withholding of physician billing for inappropriate prescribing
Restriction	Physical environment—opportunity Social environment—opportunity	Limit initiating of antipsychotic prescribing to specialists (e.g., psychiatrists) via the provincial formulary

(Continued)

TABLE 7.2 Intervention Functions with Potential Examples Related to Antipsychotic Prescribing—cont'd

Intervention	Potential Model of Behavior Addressed (Michie, Ashford, et al., 2011; Michie, van Stralen, et al., 2011)	Examples of Potential Strategies Related to Antipsychotic Prescribing
Environmental restructuring	Automatic—motivation Physical environment— opportunity Social environment—opportunity	Use on-screen prompts in computerized decision-support systems to guide appropriate selection and/or antipsychotic monitoring
Modeling	Automatic—motivation	Use video clips demonstrating psychiatrists' clinical assessments, prescribing, and monitoring of antipsychotics
Enablement	Psychological ability—capability Physical ability—capability Physical environment— opportunity Social environment—opportunity Automatic—motivation	Providing general practitioners with access to psychiatrists and pharmacists for advice and guidance on patient cases

Not surprisingly, education and training are very commonly used intervention functions aimed at changing the behavior of prescribers, following the theory that if prescribers know and are shown how to do something correctly, they will do it. Decades of research regarding changing human behaviors, such as those for healthy eating and reducing unhealthy lifestyle choices, point to the limited effectiveness of education and training when used in isolation of other intervention functions. We regularly use education and training in our roles as researchers, teachers, and program developers, but we do so in conjunction with other intervention functions, typically with positive results, as discussed later. We believe, from our own experiences, which align with a large body of research, that knowledge alone does not beget change.

In our consideration of how to move antipsychotic prescribing in youth toward a more evidence-informed practice, policy directions from relevant clinical and regulatory or oversight bodies are also relevant. For example, the American Psychiatric Association Choosing Wisely campaign includes one of five key messages: "Don't routinely prescribe antipsychotic medications as a first-line intervention for children and adolescents for any diagnosis other than psychotic disorders" (American Psychiatric Association, 2014). There also exist clinical guidelines (Kendall, Hollis, Stafford, Taylor, & Guideline Development Group, 2013; Pilling et al., 2013) for conditions in which antipsychotics are often prescribed to children and youth, as well as other prescribing and monitoring guides specifically related to antipsychotics and their adverse effects (Chehil & Kutcher, 2007; Gardner & Teehan, 2011; Ho et al., 2011; Pringsheim, Panagiotopoulos, Davidson, Ho, & CAMESA Guideline Group, 2011). Service provider policies and therapeutic guidelines are especially relevant, given that antipsychotic prescribing is part of service delivery and this can vary across provider organizations (e.g., hospitals, juvenile justice settings).

When further examining the various interventions that may be included it is important to examine the evidence of that intervention's impact. A useful resource for evidence on various intervention functions and behavior change techniques (BCTs) can be found in the Canadian Agency for Drugs and Technologies in Health Rx for Change database (CADTH Rx) (see Appendix A). This database informs whether certain interventions (e.g., education, training, incentivization, persuasion) and BCTs (e.g., audit and feedback, action planning, motivational interviewing) are effective in changing prescribing practices and if there may be differences in effectiveness across various intervention options (e.g., to what extent does incentivization change behavior as compared to coercion?).

SELECTION OF BEHAVIOR CHANGE TECHNIQUES

The final step (Table 7.1) in designing interventions for behavior change involves selecting various BCTs that bring about the desired effect (Abraham & Michie, 2008; Michie, Ashford, et al., 2011; Michie, van Stralen, et al., 2011; Michie et al., 2013). There are numerous potential BCTs to use, and a review of all potential strategies is beyond the scope of this chapter. For example, audit and feedback have been used to influence physician prescribing; there are over 45 reviews on this topic. We use the next section to describe some of our own experiences and ideas with reference to BCTs applied to improving psychotropic prescribing.

EXAMPLES OF INTERVENTION FUNCTIONS AND BEHAVIOR CHANGE TECHNIQUES FOR IMPROVING USE OF ANTIPSYCHOTICS

Some of the interventions that we have used with pre-licensure and post-licensure healthcare professionals include education, training, and modeling. We have developed and applied these interventions based on our reading of the peer-reviewed and gray literatures as well as the experiential knowledge obtained and enhanced as we have engaged in these interventions. We recognize that our approach, as clinicians and educators, has evolved over time as we have experienced feedback from prescribers and have had the opportunity to observe changes in prescribing trends and philosophies of those with whom we have worked. Spanning two decades of working with prescribers of psychotropics in youth, we have noted a number of issues common across our interventions that need to be addressed. Examples of these include: balancing prescriber experience and authority with increasing patient and family expectations of shared decision making; balancing responsibilities for decision making and management of treatment process between youth and parents or caregivers; and balancing decision making between youth and parents or caregivers while maintaining the privacy and confidentiality of all parties (Kutcher & McLuckie, 2010).

A core component of our interventions, such as education and training sessions, is making clear to prescribers and patients alike the importance of the need to set treatment goals and manage medicine-related treatment outcome expectations for both the benefits and risks of treatment. From a clinical perspective, there are four main illness- and medication-related objectives that prescribers and patients need to clearly address when using antipsychotic medicines, regardless of the specific indication or the specific medication at issue: (1) improve symptoms the person is experiencing, (2) improve functioning and promote return to regular responsibilities and activities, (3) prevent relapse of symptoms and dysfunction, and (4) minimize or avoid medication-related adverse effects throughout the treatment course. The importance of prescribers and patients (young people and parents/caretakers) working together to clearly identify these objectives and operationalize them cannot be overstated. For example: What does it mean to have symptom improvement? Which symptoms? How much improvement? When can this be expected? What should be done if expected outcomes are not achieved? And so on. For each of the four objectives it is essential to identify and manage expectations, apply effective techniques to monitor outcomes (both therapeutic success and untoward outcomes), and decide what to do in case of adverse reactions (see Chapter 4). To help ensure that our efforts, including those dedicated to education, training, and modeling, actually lead to improved behaviors in clinicians, several additional BCTs are required and examples are provided in Table 7.3.

IMPLEMENTATION OF INTERVENTIONS TO CHANGE BEHAVIORS

Once the intervention is designed based on the stepwise approach outlined earlier, the implementation process occurs. This is when we reflect on, map, and characterize factors related to the inner and outer contexts of prescribing using the CFIR (Figure 7.3). Ongoing monitoring of the impact of behavioral change interventions for changing prescribing practices is also necessary to ensure that desired changes are maintained over time. Recently, Chambers, Glasgow, and Stange (2013) debated important considerations regarding "program drift," in which program or protocol deviations lead to a decrease in the expected benefits to patients over time, and "voltage drop," which refers to the loss of expected effect as interventions go from efficacy to effectiveness and from small and controlled environments to broad-based and widespread implementation

TABLE 7.3 Behavior Change Techniques (Michie, Ashford, et al., 2011; Michie, van Stralen, et al., 2011) to Address Behavior Change in Prescribing and Monitoring of Antipsychotics

Behavior Change Technique	Examples of Strategies Used
Provide information on consequences of behavior in general	Discuss pharmacoepidemiologic evidence regarding antipsychotic prescription trends, evidence for effectiveness, and information on risks
Provide information about others' approval	Use contact-based education with people with lived experience of mental illnesses to discuss what experiences have been positive and negative related to current prescribing trends
Provide normative information about others' behaviors	Discuss best practice and what psychiatrists do for gold-standard prescribing and monitoring of antipsychotics
Facilitate social comparisons	Show trends in prescribing and monitoring locally, nationally, and internationally for comparisons
Goal setting (behavior)	Encourage prescribers to make resolutions, such as increasing monitoring of people prescribed antipsychotics
Action planning	Help clinicians to develop SMART (specific, measurable, achievable, relevant, time-bound) goals around increasing monitoring of antipsychotic treatments
Provide instruction on how to perform the behavior	Tell and show clinicians how to monitor for antipsychotic-related side effects through case-based learning
Model/demonstrate the behavior	Use a simulated patient, typically a trained actor using information from a peer-reviewed case/scenario developed by those with clinical expertise, interacting with a clinician to demonstrate the techniques for assessing when antipsychotics are required and for monitoring antipsychotic side effects. Show how to use monitoring forms
Teach to use prompts/cues	Put a copy of monitoring forms on walls next to computers capable of e-prescribing or next to prescription pads. Ask office support staff to flag and mark charts of people receiving antipsychotics

(Continued)

TABLE 7.3 Behavior Change Techniques (Michie, Ashford, et al., 2011; Michie, van Stralen, et al., 2011) to Address Behavior Change in Prescribing and Monitoring of Antipsychotics—cont'd

Behavior Change Technique	Examples of Strategies Used
Use of follow-up prompts	Use letters and telephone calls to prescribers regarding monitoring
Prompt practice	Encourage prescribers to rehearse and repeat monitoring activities with all patients
Environmental restructuring	Use computerized-reminders through electronic medical records or decision-support tools to prompt physicians to use monitoring and reevaluation of therapy and youth goals
Time management	Teach clinicians how to examine their workflow and look for efficiency opportunities that enable more time for assessment and monitoring

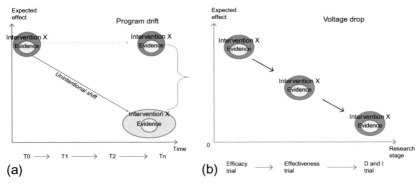

FIGURE 7.7 Program drift and voltage drop related to intervention implementation. T0, T1, Tn represent the progression of time; D is dissemination and I is implementation. From Chambers et al. (2013), BioMed Central, Implementation Science.

(Figure 7.7). A good example of these phenomena in clinical practice is when an intervention is implemented and changes are made so that it fits the context of the environment and practitioners. This adaptability of the intervention is necessary for its broad uptake. In the case of guidelines, for example, monitoring certain blood levels at specific intervals is recommended when initiating or continuing prescriptions for antipsychotics. Prescribers may alter the recommended frequency and kinds of blood work to be collected depending on patient access to blood collection facilities, the cost of testing, acceptability of blood collection to families, physician capability and motivation for assessing and monitoring repeated blood work (which may be based on experiences with other patients prescribed the same medicine), and so on. Prescribers may also alter their adherence to guideline-concordant monitoring for continued prescribing when there is less certainty regarding what to do with the results of a test. An example with antipsychotic use is prolactin levels. Although there are recommendations around monitoring, this lab value can often be elevated in youth taking antipsychotics with or without clinical symptoms (e.g., lactation, irregular menses). It is in youth without clinical symptoms that the difficulty arises, regarding what steps are to be taken once an elevated level is found. This may encourage an inertia and uncertainty, leading clinicians to decrease lab-based monitoring and focus on clinical symptoms, thus deviating from guideline-concordant monitoring.

Chambers and colleagues proposed that we conceptualize intervention implementation in a Dynamic Sustainability Framework (Figure 7.8) (Chambers et al., 2013). This framework describes maximizing the fit of interventions between practice settings and the broader ecological system through continued learning and problem solving, ongoing intervention adaptation considering fit with multilevel contexts, and ongoing improvements. Practically, some of this may be accomplished through ongoing monitoring, ongoing education, and ongoing clinician support via face-to-face or electronic interfaces. This also means that we must consider flexibility in intervention design and the implications of evaluation methods for interventions as a whole or in their component parts which undergo adaptation. This means that interventions aimed at improving antipsychotic prescribing will not only require substantial effort in terms of implementation and impact evaluation, but will also require substantial effort to ensure sustainability and adaptation as evidence changes and evolves. For example, if a group or organization developed electronic clinical tools integrated within an electronic health record decision-

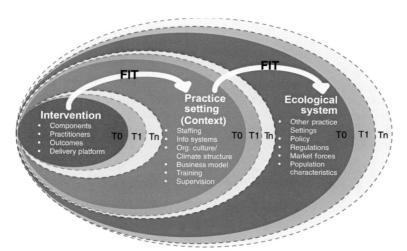

FIGURE 7.8 The Dynamic Sustainability Framework. T0, T1, Tn represent the progression of time. From Chambers et al. (2013), BioMed Central, Implementation Science.

support, a sustainability process, distinct from the implementation phase, will be required. The sustainability process and evaluation piece will likely require attention and consideration directed at factors including but not limited to changes in the practice setting including the practice panel (e.g., number and type of patients) and clinic staff (e.g., clinical, administrative) and changes in the broader health system. For the example of prolactin levels given earlier, as more evidence becomes available, there may be enhanced clarity about the frequency of monitoring and establishment of important cutoffs for prolactin levels in the absence of clinical symptoms. The intervention (i.e., the monitoring guidelines) that undergoes modification to reflect current evidence will drive changes in the sustainability planning so that new evidence and findings impacting the intervention may be integrated and adapted.

FUTURE CONSIDERATIONS

We have discussed several areas in which research is needed to explore patient-physician relationships surrounding the use of antipsychotic medicine and other psychotropic decision making in prescribing so that optimization of care outcomes can occur. This is a multifarious phenomenon that not only requires a systematic approach to designing evidence-informed behavior change interventions for individuals (prescribers) but must also consider the behaviors of youth and families in their use of the health system. These latter two considerations in particular have not been addressed conceptually or operationally to date. A comprehensive examination of the contexts in which all behaviors occur is also warranted but is complicated by the fact that environments and sociocultural contexts are varied and often nonreplicable across settings and even within one setting over time. The relative impacts of these factors on desired outcomes must also be determined. For example, are cultural factors as or more important than individual experiences in the determination of medication use? When considering changing the behaviors of individuals regarding antipsychotic prescribing for children and youth much more work is needed, especially to determine which BCTs, intervention functions, and policy categories not only provide effective improvements in prescribing and monitoring but are also adaptable to changing circumstances as time progresses and new knowledge is gained, translated, and disseminated.

REFERENCES

Abraham, C., & Michie, S. (2008). A taxonomy of behavior change techniques used in interventions. *Health Psychology*, 27(3), 379–387. http://dx.doi.org/10.1037/0278-6133.27.3.379.

American Psychiatric Association. (2014). Choosing wisely: Five things physicians and patients should question. Retrieved 03/07/2014 from http://www.choosingwisely.org/doctor-patient-lists/american-psychiatric-association/.

Canadian Standards Association. (2013). *Psychological health and safety in the workplace—Prevention, promotion and guidance to staged implementation.* No. CAN/CSA-Z1003-13/BNQ 9700-803/2013.

Cane, J., O'Connor, D., & Michie, S. (2012). Validation of the theoretical domains framework for use in behaviour change and implementation research. *Implementation Science, 7*, 37. http://dx.doi.org/10.1186/1748-5908-7-37.

Chambers, D. A., Glasgow, R. E., & Stange, K. C. (2013). The dynamic sustainability framework: Addressing the paradox of sustainment amid ongoing change. *Implementation Science, 8*, 117. http://dx.doi.org/10.1186/1748-5908-8-117.

Charles, C., Gafni, A., & Whelan, T. (1999). Decision-making in the physician-patient encounter: Revisiting the shared treatment decision-making model. *Social Science & Medicine (1982), 49*(5), 651–661.

Chehil, S., & Kutcher, S. (2007). *Mental health therapeutic outcomes tool (TOT)*. Retrieved from http://teenmentalhealth.org/toolbox/mental-health-therapeutic-outcomes-tool-tot/.

Craig, P., Dieppe, P., Macintyre, S., Michie, S., Nazareth, I., Petticrew, M., et al. (2008). Developing and evaluating complex interventions: The new medical research council guidance. *BMJ, 337*, a1655. http://dx.doi.org/10.1136/bmj.a1655.

Damschroder, L. J., Aron, D. C., Keith, R. E., Kirsh, S. R., Alexander, J. A., & Lowery, J. C. (2009). Fostering implementation of health services research findings into practice: A consolidated framework for advancing implementation science. *Implementation Science, 4*, 50. http://dx.doi.org/10.1186/1748-5908-4-50.

Einarson, T. R. (2005). The Authority/Pharmacotherapy care model: An explanatory model of the drug use process in primary care. *Research in Social & Administrative Pharmacy, 1*(1), 101–117. http://dx.doi.org/10.1016/j.sapharm.2004.12.003.

Floersch, J., Townsend, L., Longhofer, J., Munson, M., Winbush, V., Kranke, D., et al. (2009). Adolescent experience of psychotropic treatment. *Transcultural Psychiatry, 46*(1), 157–179. http://dx.doi.org/10.1177/1363461509102292.

Gardner, D. M., & Teehan, M. D. (2011). *Antipsychotics and their side effects*. Cambridge, England: Cambridge University Press.

Hamann, J., Leucht, S., & Kissling, W. (2003). Shared decision making in psychiatry. *Acta Psychiatrica Scandinavica, 107*(6), 403–409.

Hamann, J., Mendel, R., Buhner, M., Kissling, W., Cohen, R., Knipfer, E., et al. (2012). How should patients behave to facilitate shared decision making—The doctors' view. *Health Expectations, 15*(4), 360–366. http://dx.doi.org/10.1111/j.1369-7625.2011.00682.x.

Hamann, J., Mendel, R., Cohen, R., Heres, S., Ziegler, M., Buhner, M., et al. (2009). Psychiatrists' use of shared decision making in the treatment of schizophrenia: Patient characteristics and decision topics. *Psychiatric Services, 60*(8), 1107–1112. http://dx.doi.org/10.1176/appi.ps.60.8.1107.

Hendriks, A. M., Jansen, M. W., Gubbels, J. S., De Vries, N. K., Paulussen, T., & Kremers, S. P. (2013). Proposing a conceptual framework for integrated local public health policy, applied to childhood obesity—The behavior change ball. *Implementation Science, 8*, 46. http://dx.doi.org/10.1186/1748-5908-8-46.

Ho, J., Panagiotopoulos, C., McCrindle, B., Grisaru, S., & Pringsheim, T. CAMESA Guideline Group. (2011). Management recommendations for metabolic complications associated with second generation antipsychotic use in children and youth. *Journal of the Canadian Academy of Child and Adolescent Psychiatry, 20*(3), 234–241.

Kendall, T., Hollis, C., Stafford, M., & Taylor, C., & Guideline Development Group. (2013). Recognition and management of psychosis and schizophrenia in children and young people: Summary of NICE guidance. *BMJ, 346*, f150. http://dx.doi.org/10.1136/bmj.f150.

Kutcher, S. (2011). Facing the challenge of care for child and youth mental health in Canada: A critical commentary, five suggestions for change and a call to action. *Healthcare Quarterly, 14*(2), 14–21.

Kutcher, S., & McLuckie, A. (2010). *Evergreen: A child and youth mental health framework for Canada.* Calgary, AB: Mental Health Commission of Canada.

Kutcher, S., & McLuckie, A. (2011). Evergreen: A child and youth mental health framework for Canada. *Paediatrics & Child Health, 16*(7), 388.

Kutcher, S., & Wei, Y. (2014). School mental health literacy: A national curriculum guide shows promising results. *Education Canada, 54*(2).

Kutcher, S., Wei, Y., & Weist, M. (Eds.). (in press). *International school mental health for adolescents—global opportunities and challenges.* Cambridge, UK: Cambridge University Press.

Longhofer, J., & Floersch, J. (2010). Desire and disappointment: Adolescent psychotropic treatment and adherence. *Anthropology & Medicine, 17*(2), 159–172. http://dx.doi.org/10.1080/136484 70.2010.493599.

Malpass, A., Shaw, A., Sharp, D., Walter, F., Feder, G., Ridd, M., et al. (2009). "Medication career" or "moral career"? The two sides of managing antidepressants: A meta-ethnography of patients' experience of antidepressants. *Social Science & Medicine (1982), 68*(1), 154–168. http://dx.doi.org/10.1016/j.socscimed.2008.09.068.

Metge, C., & Sketris, I. S. (2007). Pharmaceutical policy. In N. J. MacKinnon (Ed.), *Safe and effective: The eight essential elements of an optimal medication-use system* (pp. 117–158). Ottawa: Canadian Pharmacists Association.

Michie, S., Ashford, S., Sniehotta, F. F., Dombrowski, S. U., Bishop, A., & French, D. P. (2011). A refined taxonomy of behaviour change techniques to help people change their physical activity and healthy eating behaviours: The CALO-RE taxonomy. *Psychology & Health, 26*(11), 1479–1498. http://dx.doi.org/10.1080/08870446.2010.540664.

Michie, S., Fixsen, D., Grimshaw, J. M., & Eccles, M. P. (2009). Specifying and reporting complex behaviour change interventions: The need for a scientific method. *Implementation Science, 4,* 40. http://dx.doi.org/10.1186/1748-5908-4-40.

Michie, S., Richardson, M., Johnston, M., Abraham, C., Francis, J., Hardeman, W., et al. (2013). The behavior change technique taxonomy (v1) of 93 hierarchically clustered techniques: Building an international consensus for the reporting of behavior change interventions. *Annals of Behavioral Medicine,* http://dx.doi.org/10.1007/s12160-013-9486-6.

Michie, S., van Stralen, M. M., & West, R. (2011). The behaviour change wheel: A new method for characterising and designing behaviour change interventions. *Implementation Science, 6,* 42. http://dx.doi.org/10.1186/1748-5908-6-42.

Moses, T. (2011). Adolescents' commitment to continuing psychotropic medication: A preliminary investigation of considerations, contradictions, and correlates. *Child Psychiatry and Human Development, 42*(1), 93–117. http://dx.doi.org/10.1007/s10578-010-0209-y.

Murphy, A. L., Gardner, D. M., Kisely, S., Cooke, C., Kutcher, S. P., & Hughes, J. (2015). A qualitative study of antipsychotic medication experiences in youth. *Journal of the Canadian Academy of Child and Adolescent Psychiatry, 24*(1), 61–69.

Pilling, S., Gould, N., Whittington, C., Taylor, C., Scott, S., & Guideline Development Group. (2013). Recognition, intervention, and management of antisocial behaviour and conduct disorders in children and young people: Summary of NICE-SCIE guidance. *BMJ, 346,* f1298. http://dx.doi.org/10.1136/bmj.f1298.

Pringsheim, T., Panagiotopoulos, C., Davidson, J., Ho, J., & CAMESA Guideline Group. (2011). Evidence-based recommendations for monitoring safety of second generation antipsychotics in children and youth. *Journal of the Canadian Academy of Child and Adolescent Psychiatry, 20*(3), 218–233.

Sketris, I. S., Langille Ingram, E. M., & Lummis, H. L. (2009). Strategic opportunities for effective optimal prescribing and medication management. *The Canadian Journal of Clinical Pharmacology, 16*(1), e103–e125.

Sketris, I. S., Langille Ingram, E., Lummis, H., & Health Council of Canada (2007). *Optimal prescribing and medication use in Canada*. Toronto, ON: Health Council of Canada.

Wei, Y., Kutcher, S., & Szumilas, M. (2011). Comprehensive school mental health: An integrated "school-based pathway to care" model for Canadian secondary schools. *McGill Journal of Education*, *46*(2), 213–230.

Chapter 8

Canadian Initiatives and Recommendations: Safeguarding the Health of Children and Youth Receiving Off-Label Treatment with Antipsychotics

Nina Di Pietro, Judy Illes

National Core for Neuroethics, Division of Neurology, Faculty of Medicine, University of British Columbia, Vancouver, British Columbia, Canada

INTRODUCTION

The expert authors contributing to this volume on the use of off-label antipsychotic treatments have highlighted important areas of concern regarding young people with mental health conditions; the need for more research on safety and efficacy, standardized health monitoring across hospitals and clinics, greater awareness and monitoring of adverse reactions in patients, improvements in the availability of nonpharmacological interventions, and changes in prescribing practices that reduce off-label and polypharmacy use are among the many and emerge as top priorities. These concerns have not gone unnoticed, either in Canada and the Pacific Northwest where the author base for this volume is largely situated or in the broader international landscape of care for the mentally ill. Policy makers, federal health agencies, industry, medical associations, and academic institutions have all worked together to find solutions and address these issues. Here we take a few pages to review these efforts, identify remaining gaps, and offer recommendations on how to move forward within four key domains: (1) postapproval health and safety monitoring, (2) informed consent, (3) pediatric clinical trials, and (4) pharmaceutical industry regulation.

The Science and Ethics of Antipsychotic Use in Children. http://dx.doi.org/10.1016/B978-0-12-800016-8.00008-8

POST-APPROVAL MONITORING OF OFF-LABEL ANTIPSYCHOTIC PRESCRIPTIONS

Reporting Adverse Events

There are many benefits of prescribing drugs for unapproved indications and subgroups of the population; however, collecting safety and efficacy data is critical for detecting adverse reactions and informing decision-makers about whether or not a treatment should be started or discontinued. In 2014, the Senate's Standing Committee on Social Affairs, Science and Technology released a report to address concerns regarding off-label prescribing practices in general, where the drastic and concerning increase in the off-label use of antidepressant and antipsychotic drugs in children was emphasized. The report highlights steps taken by the federal regulatory agency, Health Canada, to try to improve knowledge of the risks and benefits associated with off-label medications prescribed to children. In particular, it highlights the partnership between Health Canada and the Canadian Paediatric Society that has led to the creation of a national surveillance program, the Canadian Paediatric Surveillance Program (CPSP), which aims to "collect safety information on drugs used in treating children from over 2500 pediatricians and pediatric subspecialists each month" (http://www.cpsp.cps.ca). One of the main goals of the program is to ensure the safety of young people through ongoing monitoring of reported adverse drug events and through subsequent public health announcements that raise awareness of emerging health and safety concerns. According to the CPSP, Health Canada received 28,675 reports of adverse drug reaction (ADR) cases in 2011; 6% of these cases involved patients under the age of 19 and antipsychotics were included in the top 10 list of health products that were associated with ADRs. In response, the CPSP issued several notices on their website regarding unwanted side effects associated with the use of second-generation antipsychotics in children and youth (see "ADR Tips of the Month" on the CPSP website at http://www.cpsp.cps.ca/publications/adr-tips-of-the-month).

Health Canada also disseminates drug safety information through an electronic subscription service that provides health product advisories by email (http://www.hc-sc.gc.ca/dhp-mps/medeff/index_e.html) and a free subscription to the *Canadian Adverse Reaction Newsletter* (*CARN*), which is published quarterly and is considered a reputable source of adverse reaction information by healthcare professionals. Furthering these efforts, the Government of Canada introduced Bill C-17, the "Protecting Canadians from Unsafe Drugs Act" (also known as Vanessa's Law) in December 2013, which requires drug companies to provide health warnings for children on medication labels and to conduct further testing on a product when safety concerns emerge. Vanessa's Law also enables the government to require mandatory ADR reporting by public healthcare institutions such as hospitals. To help implement this, Health Canada has commissioned a nonprofit organization called *Accreditation Canada* to assess the performance of many of Canada's hospitals and other health facilities on ADR reporting and to develop standards and protocols for timely documentation.

The ADR Reporting Process: Challenges and Solutions

Despite positive initiatives, healthcare providers have voiced doubts about ongoing practices for collecting and analyzing safety data and have identified gaps in the reporting system. In principle, for example, when a patient displays an unwanted side effect from a medication, the treating physician should notify Health Canada through the Canada Vigilance Program by filling out an ADR form. In reality, however, reporting is often inconsistent and unstructured, as it remains strictly voluntary for physicians who practice outside of hospitals to do so. Mandatory reporting has been proposed to address this issue, but there is a lack of consensus among policy makers and medical professionals about the effectiveness of such a policy. Critics of mandatory reporting argue that it would be difficult to implement and enforce unless user-friendly electronic reporting processes are in place and standard protocols are established (Senate's Standing Committee on Social Affairs, Science and Technology, 2014). Moreover, reporting would only be effective if data from ADR reports are analyzed promptly and health warnings issued to drug manufacturers and the Canadian public in a timely fashion. A report from the Auditor General of Canada (2011) found that Health Canada's assessment of and response to potential safety concerns was too slow; assessments can take up to 2 years and notifications to drug manufacturers to update labels can take as much as an additional 20 months. In response, the health agency has agreed to develop and implement standard operating procedures for streamlining reporting and assessment, including new formalized tracking systems.

Another challenge to safety vigilance is that information provided on ADR reports is often insufficient to determine whether or not the medication suspected of causing the ADR is being prescribed off-label (Senate's Standing Committee on Social Affairs, Science and Technology, 2014). In many cases, information such as patient age or the condition for which the medication was prescribed is missing. A recent example of this is illustrated in the April 2014 issue of the *CARN* (Bawolak, 2014), which highlights three reports of liver failure in patients taking the atypical antipsychotic drug quetiapine (Seroquel). The newsletter states that of the three cases, "one report was unassessable due to limited information." In response, the Senate's Standing Committee on Social Affairs, Science and Technology (2014) recommended that ADR forms be expanded to include information such as patient's age, pregnancy or nursing status, and the indication for which the drug is being prescribed to determine off-label status, and that this information be made mandatory.

Another recommendation is to require Canadian provinces and territories to report data related to prescription drugs via electronic medical record (EMR) systems. Several provinces already have prescription databases in place. British

Columbia, for example, has created PharmaNet, a province-wide network that links all BC pharmacies to a central database that collects information about every prescription dispensed in the province. To maximize impact, it is essential that electronic health systems are implemented on a national level and made available online to all physicians and pharmacists. Currently, such systems remain in the early stages of development. Ongoing research is needed to determine the impact of EMRs on patient safety outcomes, identify potential pitfalls (e.g., breaches in privacy, hacking), and establish common measures for healthcare professionals to determine patient safety outcomes (Canada Health Infoway, 2007). Adoption of digital health systems also requires cultural and organizational changes in healthcare delivery that take time. In recognition of this, the federal government funds initiatives such as Canada Health Infoway, which is an independent, not-for-profit organization that works with provinces and territories to integrate private and secure e-health systems into existing infrastructures and provide healthcare professionals with immediate access to complete and accurate patient information.

INFORMED CONSENT FOR PATIENTS AND CAREGIVERS

Studies have shown that parents are often uninformed about the off-label status of medications used to treat their children, despite evidence that they desire such information (Bang et al., 2014; Lenk, Koch, Zappel, & Wiesemann, 2009). Legal and health scholars have argued that this amounts to providing patients with experimental drugs without their consent (Rosoff & Coleman, 2011; Salbu, 1999). This represents an important ethical gap for patient autonomy and informed consent. Patient advocates recommend that consumers be given access to information about drug licensing status and about ADRs through the creation of patient information leaflets that would accompany all prescription drugs when dispensed at the pharmacy and that would include information on how to report an ADR to Health Canada, either online or through a national ADR-reporting telephone hotline (Senate's Standing Committee on Social Affairs, Science and Technology, 2014). Others propose that physicians should also notify patients when a drug is being prescribed off-label, either in person or by indicating it on the prescription, and that they obtain informed consent from patients before issuing the script (Haw & Stubbs, 2005). There are several caveats to this approach, however. For one, physicians may be unaware that they are prescribing an antipsychotic drug off-label. According to a study by Chen, Wynia, Moloney, and Alexander (2009), 19% of physicians mistakenly believed that the antipsychotic quetiapine is approved for the treatment of dementia with agitation. Proposed explanations for this disconnect included lack of time and lack of access to resources for physicians to keep up-to-date with emerging clinical trial evidence and FDA approvals. This is especially challenging in the field of psychiatry, where there is particular difficulty establishing the boundaries of evidence and medications are frequently used off-label for clinical innovation (Kuehn, 2010).

To increase awareness and help doctors with decision-making, we suggest that tools such as electronic databases that record patient and prescription data also be used to automatically signal doctors when a script is off-label or comes with a health warning. A standardized patient consent form outlining the known risks and benefits of the medication should accompany this information. No doubt, uptake of a formal consent process by healthcare professionals would be challenging. In a survey of 427 Canadian psychiatrists from the province of Ontario, for example, psychiatrists were more reluctant to disclose adverse re-action information when the antipsychotic medication was prescribed for acute care (i.e., for less than 3 months or in an emergency situation) and voiced concerns about the impact of risk disclosure on patient compliance with taking the medication. This significant finding emerged even while almost all respondents believed that competent patients or substitute decision makers of incompetent patients should be informed about the benefits and risks of antipsychotic medications (Schachter & Kleinman, 2004). In a follow-up study of the same cohort, Schachter and Kleinman (2006) reported that 63% of psychiatrists documented the informed consent process in patient charts but felt that obtaining formal signed consent forms from patients was unnecessary. Further research is needed to identify the reasons behind this reluctance.

Informed Consent Involving Minors

Prescribing a psychotropic medication to a minor presents special ethical challenges and considerations throughout the consent process. In the decision to medicate, several actors are involved: the child patient, the legal caregiver, and in part, but not insignificantly, other individuals who may have influence, such as the treating physician, teachers, other family members, and social workers (see also Chapter 7 by Murphy et al.).

Complex interactions between these actors can both facilitate and impede the process of obtaining valid consent for psychopharmacological treatment of children. In cases where a child or adolescent is involved in giving assent, Krener and Mancina (1994) propose that at least five factors be considered by the prescriber: (1) the rights of the child, (2) the child's relationships to the adults responsible for his or her care, (3) the child's developmental capacity to understand the treatment, (4) the process of consent as it unfolds within the treatment alliance, and (5) the potential for coercion of the minor, either by adults in the environment or by "therapeutic coercion" in circumstances when treatment is determined to be the only option. In the ideal situation, the physician should become acquainted with the minor's wishes, understandings, and any points of ambivalence about the decision to medicate by providing a safe space for their expression (Krener & Mancina, 1994). In cases where the minor has difficulties communicating wishes—due to anything from shyness to an underlying developmental condition such as autism—the parent must assume a greater role in helping with translation and interpretation. Furthermore, children with externalizing conduct disorders or oppositional/defiant symptoms may also experience coercion because of the inherent emotional strains placed on the parent-child relationship (Krener & Mancina, 1994). Other barriers to a successful informed consent process include: (1) incomplete knowledge about the safety and efficacy profiles of the medication, (2) lack of physician experience with use of the drug, (3) insufficient communication about risks and benefits to patients, caregivers, or both, (4) pressure or coercion of patient or caregiver to consent to treatment (e.g., legal, school, or social pressures), and (5) lack of compliance (e.g., consent by caregiver is given but patient refuses to take medication or parent refuses to give medication).

Yet other important factors include changing attitudes toward the decision to medicate based on experiences with the medications, such as unwanted side effects, and changes in the developmental capacity of the minor as she/he matures and becomes more involved in the decision-making process. A good demonstration of this is found in the work of Murphy et al. (2013), who interviewed prescribers, parents, and children about their experiences with antipsychotic-related weight gain over time. Here, Murphy et al. quote a parent, "… Then she started to gain some weight with the Invega… And gaining weight just wasn't in the cards. And she was really quite upset by that… The barriers really are around the weight gain and then they don't want to stay on it." In time, knowledge about the efficacy and safety of the medication may change, as evidence emerges from clinical studies or as prescribers become more experienced with prescribing the drug, causing a reluctance to prescribe a particular antipsychotic or leading a patient to withdraw from treatment. Again, Murphy et al. (2013) effectively demonstrate this. A prescriber they interviewed stated, "I tend to stay away from olanzapine because I've had experience and …, I tend to use quetiapine. That is such a crap shoot … This is more like the art or the cookery, the recipe of medicine, but I've had experience with clients becoming diabetic on olanzapine." Hence, consent is a fluid process that must be regularly revisited with patients and families.

INCENTIVIZING CLINICAL TRIALS AND EXPANDING THE KNOWLEDGE BASE

Clinical trials are essential to establish the effectiveness of antipsychotics for off-label uses, determine proper dosing, and identify what side effects may occur, if any. Historically, clinical trials have excluded children from participating because of concerns over real or perceived potential harms to such a vulnerable group (see Chapter 5 by McGlanaghy, Di Pietro, and Wilfond for more on this). As a result, the vast majority of pharmaceutical products are not designed specifically for use in children. It is now understood that this is problematic. The lack of involvement of young people in clinical trials has led to a dearth of information regarding the proper use, dosing, and labeling of the majority of antipsychotics available on the market, leaving physicians and families without adequate guidance to protect child health and safety.

The Canadian Clinical Trial Landscape: Lengthy, Expensive, Complex

The only way to address lack of information is to gather more data. In recognition of the gap for children, the Canadian Institutes of Health Research has contributed $7.9 million for research related to off-label drug use over the past 5 years (Senate's Standing Committee on Social Affairs, Science and Technology, 2014). Nonetheless, pediatric clinical trials for antipsychotics still lag behind, especially in Canada, where only 3.4% of pediatric trials for antipsychotics are registered (see Chapter 5 by McGlanaghy and Wilfond). Recent data indicate that Canadian clinical trial activity and spending on research and development (R&D) has dropped overall. Canada's share of clinical trial sites sponsored by industry fell from 5% of the global total in 2005 to 4% in 2010. This corresponds to a 16% decline in the number of Canadian sites participating in clinical trials, along with fewer participants enrolled by Canadian researchers (McAllister, 2012). Industry Canada (2012) reports that from 2001 to 2012 overall R&D spending by pharmaceutical companies fell by 15.6%; in 2001, R&D expenditures totaled $1.06 billion but by 2012 they had fallen to $0.89 billion (although a 2014 survey by Canada's Research-Based Pharmaceutical Companies, reported an additional $221 million in expenditures in 2012). This decline in R&D activities seems unwarranted, given that pharmaceutical sales nearly doubled during that same time period. In 2013, total pharmaceutical sales in Canada amounted to $21.6 billion, with 89% sold to retail drug stores and 11% sold to hospitals. Government covered 42% of drug expenditures while private payers (private coverage and individuals) covered the remaining 58%. Canadian sales data indicate that drugstore sales for antipsychotics amounted to $682 million in 2012/2013; the majority (68%) were covered under provincial drug plans, making antipsychotics one of the most publicly subsidized drug classes in Canada (Morgan et al., 2013). Although data for off-label prescription sales are not available, the *Canadian Rx Atlas* reported that 4% of sales were for patients under 18 years of age.

If clinical trial data were to emerge that these medications are not as effective or as safe for children as for adults, greater regulation and labeling changes prohibiting antipsychotic use in this population would be needed and would impact government and private health insurance coverage for antipsychotic treatment. The result would be a significant revenue loss for companies. Globally, off-label uses account for up to 65% of all antipsychotic prescriptions (Sugarman, Mitchell, Frogley, Dickens, & Picchioni, 2013). Given evidence that the number of off-label antipsychotic prescriptions continues to rise (see Chapter 2 by Ortega and Pringsheim), there is little incentive for pharmaceutical companies to conduct lengthy and expensive studies that may not necessarily yield results in their favor. This concern was echoed by the Senate's Standing Committee on Social Affairs, Science and Technology (2012), which indicated that vulnerable groups are often excluded from industry-sponsored trials because they may not respond as well to drug treatment, therefore reducing the measure of a drug's effectiveness.

In addition to the potential loss in sales revenue, the process of obtaining modifications to a product license is lengthy, expensive, and complex. According to a report in the *Canadian Medical Association Journal*, "Canada is the most expensive country [in which to conduct trials], one of the slowest to initiate trials and not very efficient in terms of [patient] recruitment" (Vogel, 2011). The average cost of recruiting patients in Canada is among the highest in the world: over $17,000 per patient (Leclerc, Laberge, & Marion, 2012). Moreover, each province has distinct ethical requirements and privacy laws that make multisite research difficult.

Becoming a Leader in Pediatric Clinical Trials: Canadian Solutions

In 2011, a National Clinical Trials Summit was held to address the problem of declining clinical trial activity in Canada. Recommendations for an action plan included: (i) streamlining the ethics review process, (ii) developing a database of clinical trial registries, (iii) creating a national patient recruitment strategy, (iv) optimizing intellectual property protection policies, and (v) promoting tax credits to offset the cost of trials. In addition to these measures, others have urged stricter legislation, such as requirements for drug manufacturers to conduct post-approval studies and approval of new drugs only if clinical trials have been performed in the same population that is reasonably expected to consume the drug once it is on the market (Senate's Standing Committee on Social Affairs, Science and Technology, 2012). At the time of this book publication, however, these measures have not been implemented, perhaps due to the lack of financial support and infrastructure to implement such endeavors.

Meanwhile, to cut down on lengthy and complex application processes, several organizations are working to coordinate ethics review decisions on a national level. A leader in this area is the Maternal Infant Child, Youth Research Network (MICYRN), which is working to implement a Canadian national federated ethics review process that includes the development of a national application and consent form template and a review of privacy and ethics board legislative differences across provinces. Since 2009, Health Canada has also been working with a Pediatric Expert Advisory Committee to obtain expert advice on broad strategic issues relating to the discovery, testing, and approval of health products for children and nursing or pregnant women, including the ongoing monitoring of the safety and effectiveness of products once they are approved by Health Canada and made available on the market. A key role of the Advisory Committee is to identify opportunities within Canada's regulatory framework to encourage safe and ethical pediatric clinical trials. Here, it has suggested that Canada's Drug Safety and Effectiveness Network (DSEN) implement a strategy to conduct studies in vulnerable subgroups of the population that uses its research networks to maximize participant enrollment (DSEN coordinates a national network of over 150 researchers committed to post-market drug safety and effectiveness research).

Broadening the Scope of Evidence

Other proposed strategies to increase the evidence base for off-label prescriptions include broadening the scope of evidence beyond the gold standard in research, which involves lengthy and expensive randomized control trials (RCTs), to include alternative research methods. Proponents of this measure argue that RCTs have limited external validity because they are by design conducted under highly controlled conditions that may not reflect real world settings and may take several years to complete (Victora, Habicht, & Bryce, 2004; West et al., 2008). For ethical and other reasons, many investigators have already turned to alternative types of research methodologies and trial designs to speed innovation and deliver effective treatment options to patients (Deveaugh-Geiss et al., 2006). Table 8.1 outlines examples of these strategies. Each of the methods listed has unique strengths and weaknesses, and although the methods may not be as stringent or reliable as RCTs they can provide sufficient information about the real-world effectiveness and safety of antipsychotics to inform clinical practice.

In support of alternative approaches, a report from the Cochrane Collaboration (Anglemyer, Horvath, & Bero, 2014) concluded that the pooled outcomes of observational studies are sufficiently similar to those of RCTs, regardless of specific observational study design, and that study design is not the leading factor in determining outcomes (Anglemyer et al., 2014). Conveniently, the infrastructure for conducting these types of studies is already available in DSEN, which includes a group of researchers dedicated to understanding drug effects through observational studies. The establishment of large, multicenter trials conducted via existing clinical trials networks such as DSEN would constitute a major step forward, as they would provide sufficient power to allow the establishment of safety databases and identify moderators of treatment outcome (March et al., 2005).

CANADIAN PHARMACEUTICAL MARKETING REGULATORY POLICIES

Pharmaceutical companies play a vital role in healthcare. They invest tremendous amounts of money in research, development and marketing. It is through marketing, that healthcare providers and patients can be influenced into prescribing or wanting these medications.

James Rhee, 2009.

Physician knowledge about pharmaceutical products is often derived from pharmaceutical sales representatives whose primary goal is to promote their product while also providing information (Chalkley, 2009; Fugh-Berman & Ahari, 2007). While many physicians make decisions about off-label prescribing only after reviewing the existing literature (Senate's Standing Committee

TABLE 8.1 Examples of Clinical Trial Design Strategies; Strengths and Weaknesses

Trial Design Strategy	Design Features Pros/Cons
Double-blind randomized control trials (RCTs)	Participants are allocated at random to receive one of several clinical interventions. Patients and researchers are unaware of the allocated treatment group until the study is completed
	All groups are treated identically except for the type of experimental treatment received. One group receives a placebo (control group)
	Pros:
	Has the highest internal validity because any significant differences between groups in the outcome analysis can be attributed to the intervention and not to some other unidentified factor
	Cons:
	May not be appropriate for the assessment of interventions that have rare outcomes or effects that take a long time to develop
	May not be feasible because of financial constraints, low compliance rates, or high dropout rates
	Sibbald and Roland (1998)
Active controlled non-inferiority (or superiority) trials	Participants are guaranteed to receive a treatment. Used in instances where placebo controls may ethically need to be ruled out
	Pros:
	Ethically superior to RCTs when faced with clear evidence of efficacy for an existing standard treatment (i.e., it would be ethically unacceptable to proceed with a placebo or inactive control group in the evaluation of a new treatment for the same condition)
	Cons:
	Use of non-inferiority trials, with a less than convincing active control treatment, may potentially lead to the adoption of ineffective treatments
	Pocock (2003)

TABLE 8.1 Examples of Clinical Trial Design Strategies; Strengths and Weaknesses—cont'd

Trial Design Strategy	Design Features Pros/Cons
Adaptive	Changes can be made to trial procedures in ongoing studies, such as re-estimating the sample size or adjusting dose or study endpoints, following significant positive or negative results at interim analysis *Pros*: Flexible and efficient, which is especially useful in early clinical development Allows for prematurely stopping a trial due to safety, futility/efficacy, or both, with the option of additional adaptations based on results of interim analysis *Cons*: Overall type I error rate (i.e., rejecting the null hypothesis when it is in fact true) may be inflated when there is a shift in the target patient population Chow and Chang (2008)
Group sequential analysis	Sample size is not fixed in advance and sampling continues unless a significant positive result is obtained. If the null hypothesis is not rejected following a pre-determined maximum number of interim analyses (i.e., stopping rules), the trial is discontinued *Pros*: A conclusion may be reached at an earlier stage than would be possible with traditional RCTs, lowering the financial and human cost of trials *Cons*: Clinical trials that stop early because of evidence of therapeutic benefit are prone to exaggerate the magnitude of treatment effect Stallard (2011)
Patient preference RCTs	Patients with treatment preferences are allowed their desired treatment without being assigned to a random group, while those who do not have particular preferences are individually randomized in the usual way

Continued

TABLE 8.1 Examples of Clinical Trial Design Strategies; Strengths and Weaknesses—cont'd

Trial Design Strategy	Design Features Pros/Cons
	Pros:
	Maximizes patient recruitment and thus increases sample size
	Minimizes patient dropout or low compliance
	Cons:
	The relationship between patient preferences and the outcome of interventions is unclear but may be a source of bias, especially in patients with strong treatment preferences
	Howard and Thornicroft (2006)
Equipoise-stratified randomization	Allows participants and clinicians to choose together from a list of treatments that they prefer (based on medical factors or previous experience with a medication), which the participant would be willing to be randomly assigned to for treatment
	Pros:
	Offers maximal efficiency, giving opportunities to participate to all patients for whom there is a researchable choice of treatments
	Participants are still randomly assigned to a treatment group, minimizing chance of patient preference-related bias
	Cons:
	Can be applied only when there are multiple treatment arms that can be grouped into strata, which limits its use to a subset of clinical research studies
	Lavori et al. (2001) and Marks, Thanaseelan, and Pae (2009)
Observational studies	Allows inferences about the possible effect of a treatment when assignment of participants into a random treatment group, including a control group, is outside the control of the investigator
	Pros:
	Provides information on "real world" use and practice
	Detects signals about the benefits and risks of a treatment in the general population

TABLE 8.1 Examples of Clinical Trial Design Strategies; Strengths and Weaknesses—cont'd

Trial Design Strategy	Design Features
	Pros/Cons
	Informs future clinical practice and clinical trial hypotheses and designs in a pragmatic manner
	Cons:
	Lower validity because of difficulties in controlling levels of potential bias, confounding, and chance associations
	Jepsen, Johnsen, Gillman, and Sørensen (2004)

on Social Affairs, Science and Technology, 2014), it is unreasonable to expect prescribers to always be able to undertake exhaustive analyses. This tension of time and burden provides a window of opportunity for sales agents to influence prescribers to favor the products they are promoting (Anderson, Silverman, Loewenstein, Zinberg, & Schulkin, 2009; Fugh-Berman & Ahari, 2007; Mintzes et al., 2013; Wazana, 2000).

Industry Regulation: Policies and Pitfalls

As a general rule, drug manufacturers are prohibited from advertising their products beyond the specifics established in the product monographs approved by Health Canada. Regulation of pharmaceutical sales representatives is self-governed by industry through its national association, Canada's Research-Based Pharmaceutical Companies (Rx&D), which represents over 50 pharmaceutical companies in the country. According to the Rx&D ethical code "Members will not promote Prescription Medicines that are not approved in Canada or unauthorized uses of approved Prescription Medicines. Promotion of unauthorized Prescription Medicines and uses is prohibited irrespective of an employee's function within the Member Company" (Section 5.1.1.4). Enforcement of the code relies on each member company assigning an employee or agent to oversee compliance. Complaints filed against companies for breaches of the code are reviewed by the Industry Practices Review Committee to determine if a violation occurred. Infractions can result in monetary fines of $25,000 for the first infraction, $50,000 for a second, $75,000 for a third, and $100,000 for each subsequent violation. Moreover, penalties can be enforced through Section 31 of the Food and Drugs Act (Government of Canada, 1985), which can fine a party up to $5000 in addition to a term of imprisonment of up to 3 years for contravening the act's policies on prohibited advertising practices (Section 9.1 of the Food and Drugs Act prohibits advertising messages that discuss off-label use of a product or that neglect to mention information about potential harm). In comparison to drug sale profits, however, these financial penalties are relatively modest and do not pose a large disincentive for companies (Gibson, 2014; Rosoff & Coleman, 2011). Moreover, academic and legal experts criticize Health Canada for rarely enforcing the act in practice and have demonstrated that current approaches for regulating false claims in marketing are not working (Gibson, 2014; Mintzes et al., 2013).

To curb inappropriate practices, countries such as the United States have adopted whistleblower policies. Under the US False Claims Act, private parties may file complaints against companies. A private party that successfully demonstrates that the federal government has been defrauded through false advertising may receive up to 30% of the government's award. Since 2008, pharmaceutical companies in the United States have agreed to pay more than $13 billion to resolve Department of Justice (DOJ) allegations of fraudulent marketing practices. Notable lawsuits include a $1.4 billion fine against drug manufacturer Eli Lilly for encouraging doctors to prescribe its antipsychotic Zyprexa to children through misleading claims. The case allegedly included the distribution of a video titled "The myth of diabetes" that downplayed the risk of unwanted metabolic side effects despite evidence to the contrary (Wilson, 2010). Under the Whistleblower Act, the pharmaceutical giant Pfizer was also fined $2.3 billion for hiring child psychiatrists to help market its antipsychotic drug Geodon despite lack of approval by the FDA for pediatric use (US DOJ, 2009). Similarly, drug company AstraZeneca was fined $520 million for targeting child physicians when promoting its antipsychotic Seroquel for off-label uses to treat aggression, sleeplessness, anxiety, and depression in children (US DOJ, 2010). Most recently, Johnson & Johnson was ordered to pay a $2.2 billion fine for off-label marketing and kickbacks to doctors and pharmacists aimed at promoting the use of Risperdal in children as well as the elderly (US DOJ, 2013). To improve the enforcement of policies under the Canadian Food and Drugs Act and bolster efforts to regulate advertising practices, the Senate's Standing Committee on Social Affairs, Science and Technology (2014) recommended that similar whistlerblower policies be implemented in Canada.

Finally, one other tactic that has shown promise for reducing the effects of marketing on physician prescribing practices involves policies that restrict pharmaceutical sales representatives from interacting directly with physicians to promote drugs via sales calls or office visits, and by banning physicians from receiving gifts or sample products from sales agents (Larkin, Ang, Avorn, & Kesselheim, 2014). According to Larkin and colleagues, academic medical centers that restrict this type of activity (also referred to as "detailing" by the pharmaceutical industry) report fewer prescriptions for off-label use of promoted antidepressant and antipsychotic drugs. Interestingly, the adoption of anti-detailing policies reduced prescriptions for on-label use of promoted drugs by 34% while prescriptions for on-label use of nonpromoted drugs rose by 14% (prescriptions for off-label use of nonpromoted drugs rose by 35%). While these results suggest that restricting detailing by sales representatives may not curb off-label prescribing, they appear to promote the use of cheaper, generic drugs.

Regulation in the Age of Digital Marketing

Enforcement of marketing violations is especially challenging for regulators now that pharmaceutical companies can deliver direct-to-consumer messaging over the Internet and social media platforms. Spending for online marketing by pharmaceutical companies is projected to be in the range of USD $1.86 billion in 2015 (Gibson, 2014). In comparison to traditional print and TV media, online marketing is cost effective, reaches a bigger and broader audience, and can be used to target messages to specific groups and patient populations, including children and youth.

The task of monitoring pharmaceutical advertisements and messaging falls under the purview of the Pharmaceutical Advertising Advisory Board (PAAB), an independent Canadian agency that reviews "materials developed by pharmaceutical manufacturers predominantly for the purpose of advertising or promoting [s11] a product…" (http://www.paab.ca). Ultimately, the PAAB's goal is to ensure that any information provided about a product is evidence based and balanced. According to PAAB guidelines, websites for prescription drugs may not provide information beyond name, price, and quantity (PAAB, 2013). Legal experts claim, however, that pharmaceutical companies circumvent these restrictions by using indirect marketing strategies, such as campaigns aimed at raising awareness about a particular medical condition and encouraging patients to ask their doctor about treatment options (Gibson, 2014). A strong emphasis on messaging such as "talk to your doctor about treatment options" is often used by industry because physicians are seen by companies as the most effective way through which to generate more prescription sales of their drug product (Gibson, 2014). Given the global nature of information over the Internet, regulating online advertising requires a concerted effort from all countries. Unfortunately, Canada is not the only country faced with limited resources for such a task. Instead, Gibson (2014) suggests that government needs to step in by providing Canadian consumers with user-friendly, reliable, and neutral online health information, particularly on drug products that are approved for sale in Canada, through a single government-sponsored health information portal.

Helping Prescribers and Patients Stay Informed

In addition to online resources, medical school curricula aimed at educating physicians about pharmaceutical marketing strategies and tactics are needed. In 2013, Mintzes and colleagues published results from a research study on the experiences and opinions of primary care physicians across three countries (Canada, United States, and France) with regard to interactions with pharmaceutical sales agents who visited their offices. In all countries, physicians reported that sales agents rarely provided adequate safety information and in 13% of cases openly discussed unapproved uses for the drug they were promoting. Despite this, the majority of doctors in this study (57%) rated the scientific quality of information they received from the sales agent to be good or excellent and almost two-thirds (64%) indicated that they were more likely to begin or to increase prescribing the promoted drug following the sales visit. These findings suggest that additional training in the form of continuing medical education or medical school curricula that teach doctors how to critically evaluate and respond to drug promotion may be valuable. In an international survey conducted on behalf of the World Health Organization and others, results showed that the majority of medical school institutions provide education about drug promotion as part of the required curriculum, but that one-third of medical and one-fifth of pharmacy programs only devote 1-2 h of related training within the required curriculum (Mintzes, 2005).

Arming doctors against inappropriate marketing messages by providing them with alternative sources of information that are up to date, peer reviewed, and evidence based is critical. Such resources are woefully inadequate or missing for Canadian doctors. *Canada's Compendium of Pharmaceuticals and Specialties* (CPS), which is a primary source for information about approved drugs in Canada, does not provide any information about off-label uses. Another resource, *The Compendium of Therapeutic Choices*, provides evidence-based treatment information for more than 200 common medical conditions, including information about drug therapy during pregnancy and breastfeeding, but information about drug treatment for children and youth is limited and does not address antipsychotic use. The *Cochrane Database of Systematic Reviews* provides regular assessments of the existing research literature to establish whether or not there is acceptable evidence about the safety and efficacy of a specific treatment, but most physicians in Canada do not have full access to this $387 annual subscription-based resource. Fortunately, there is a less costly resource that health practitioners can turn to: *The Clinical Handbook of Psychotropic Drugs* (Virani, Bezchlibnyk-Butler, & Jeffries, 2011), which offers up-to-date, easy-to-use, comprehensive summaries of all the most relevant information about psychotropic drugs, including special precautions to consider when treating children and adolescents.

The establishment of independent therapeutic assessment and advisory groups in Canada may also help fill knowledge gaps. An example of such a group is the Therapeutics Initiative (TI), funded by the Ministry of Health of British Columbia. The TI aims to provide physicians and pharmacists with up-to-date, evidence-based, practical information on prescription drug therapy. Because the TI does not have ties to government, pharmaceutical industry, or other vested interest groups, it can conduct unbiased, independent, and extensive assessments of clinical evidence for distribution to physicians, pharmacists, nurses, and policy makers. Despite some successes, funding for the initiative was interrupted in 2012 due to patient privacy concerns; interruptions to drug assessments and TI activities that depend on access to patient databases have ensued. Since December 2013, however, the government has agreed to reinstate funding following the implementation of measures to enhance oversight and protection of patient information. Further investment and expansion of such initiatives is needed to arm Canadians with the best available evidence and treatment recommendations.

Finally, another avenue for countering inappropriate marketing claims that downplay unwanted side effects is to provide risk information upfront on the drug label. Since 2003, makers of atypical antipsychotics have been required by the FDA to include black box warnings on some drug labels about the risks of hyperglycemia and diabetes, including death in elderly patients taking these drugs. Labels are also required to include information about the need for glucose monitoring in patients with or at risk for diabetes. A caveat to this approach is that physician knowledge of off-label status and risk for adverse events may not be sufficient to alter prescribing practices or increase engagement in health monitoring. Uptake of health monitoring efforts for adverse reactions remains low (see Chapter 4 on by Ronsley et al.) and off-label prescriptions continue to rise (see Chapter 2 by Ortega and Pringsheim). As a result, legal experts have even argued in favor of regulating physician prescribing practices with financial penalties or license suspensions in cases where off-label use is not justified by scientific evidence and exposes patients to harm (Rosoff & Coleman, 2011). This suggestion has been met with strong opposition from the medical community, however, as it undermines the ability of physicians to exercise their professional skills and good judgment based on years of clinical experience. Such regulation would also deny the rights of patients to access off-label treatments.

SUMMARY OF GUIDELINES FOR PRESCRIBING ANTIPSYCHOTICS

Guidelines for prescribing medication off-label have been proposed by several health associations, including the Royal College of Psychiatrists (2007) and the American Psychiatric Association (2013). Taken together with the findings and proposals offered in this book, we have identified nine key recommendations for prescribers: (1) keeping up to date with evidence about the proposed drug, including possible drug interactions and potential adverse effects; (2) obtaining advice from another doctor or specialist pharmacist in cases of uncertainty; (3) disclosing to the patient or caregiver, as appropriate, when a medication is being used off-label and the known risks; (4) obtaining and documenting informed consent prior to treatment; (5) follow-up monitoring of the health of the patient at regular intervals (as outlined in Chapter 4) and revisiting consent; (6) reporting effects and adverse reactions to health agencies to increase the knowledge base (publishing data in the form of case studies is also recommended); (7) withdrawing treatment if it proves unsuccessful and providing alternatives (including sleep assessments and interventions as outlined in Chapter 6); (8) limiting concurrent antipsychotic treatments (polypharmacy); and (9) limiting the use of antipsychotics as a first-line intervention for children and adolescents with nonpsychotic disorders.

With regard to federal health agencies, our recommendations include: (1) mandating or incentivizing pharmaceutical companies to conduct pediatric clinical trials on antipsychotics targeted at the treatment of nonpsychotic disorders for which they are most often prescribed; (2) promoting non-industry-sponsored clinical trial research through increased funding opportunities and resources that support academic research and networks; (3) engaging with payers and healthcare providers to determine eligibility and reimbursement policies with respect to medications such as antipsychotics when issued for off-label use; (4) implementing e-health systems so that off-label prescribing information and adverse events can be recorded and readily shared with physicians, patients, and pharmacists; (5) creating and implementing policies that allow for better enforcement of advertising and marketing regulations; (6) implementing anti-detailing policies in medical health centers; (7) mandating that medication labeling clearly indicates off-label status and is accompanied by drug safety information leaflets; and (8) expanding funding and resources for the establishment of a national, independent, advisory group to disseminate up-to-date, evidence-based treatment recommendations for healthcare providers.

CONCLUSION

In this chapter, we have reviewed major steps taken by Health Canada and others to improve the outcomes of young Canadians receiving treatment with off-label antipsychotic medications. We have also gleaned valuable insights from our contributing authors on how researchers, healthcare professionals, and ethicists can work together to address gaps in knowledge and shortcomings in the healthcare system. We acknowledge, however, that a significant voice has been almost entirely absent from the pages of this book—the voice of patients and caregivers. Although there is no shortage of patient stories in the news media, their perspectives are conspicuously missing from the scientific and grey literature even though they have the most to gain or lose in the decision to medicate. This is an important ethical gap, as patient care and safety are now recognized as a shared responsibility, marked by a shift in patient care from doctor-driven paternalistic practices to patient-centered ones. Engagement with patients and caregivers to identify their perspectives on off-label antipsychotic prescribing practices, the provision of informed consent, ultimate treatment goals, values, and concerns, is vital to informing solutions that will work in real-life settings.

Thus, we conclude with one final recommendation: qualitative research involving young Canadians and their caregivers is needed to inform research and policy that will be adjudicated by all levels of government. It is our sincere hope that the information and perspectives represented in this book will provide much-needed context surrounding the issues related to the rise in off-label antipsychotic prescriptions, not just for healthcare professionals but also for members of the Canadian public who wish to become involved in this important conversation.

REFERENCES

American Psychiatric Association. (2013). *Five things physicians and patients should question.* Retrieved from http://www.psychiatry.org/choosingwisely.

Anderson, B. L., Silverman, G. K., Loewenstein, G. F., Zinberg, S., & Schulkin, J. (2009). Factors associated with physicians' reliance on pharmaceutical sales representatives. *Academic Medicine, 84,* 994–1002.

Anglemyer, A., Horvath, H. T., & Bero, L. (2014). Healthcare outcomes assessed with observational study designs compared with those assessed in randomized trials. *Cochrane Database of Systematic Reviews, 4,* Art. No.: MR000034. Accessed at: http://onlinelibrary.wiley.com/doi/10.1002/14651858.MR000034.pub2/abstract.

Auditor General of Canada. (2011). *Fall report on regulating pharmaceutical drugs.* Retrieved from http://www.oag-bvg.gc.ca/internet/docs/parl_oag_201111_04_e.pdf.

Bang, V., Mallad, A., Kannan, S., Bavdekar, S. B., Gogtay, N. J., & Thatte, U. M. (2014). Awareness about and views of parents on the off-label drug use in children. *The International Journal of Risk & Safety in Medicine, 26*(2), 61–70.

Bawolak, M. T. (2014). Quetiapine and acute liver failure. *Canadian Adverse Reaction Newsletter, 24*(2), 1–2.

Canada Health Infoway. (2007). *Electronic health records and patient safety: Future directions for Canada.* Retrieved from http://www.patientsafetyinstitute.ca/english/news/eventproceedings/pages/ehrroundtable.aspx.

Canada's Research-Based Pharmaceutical Companies. (2012). *Code of ethical practices.* Retrieved from http://www.canadapharma.org/home.

Canada's Research-Based Pharmaceutical Companies, Rx&D. (2014). *Summary of 2013 R&D spending and investments by Rx&D members.* Retrieved from http://www.canadapharma.org/en/our-industry.

Chalkley, P. (2009). Targeting accessible physicians. *Canadian Pharmaceutical Marketing, 2,* 29–30.

Chen, D. T., Wynia, M. K., Moloney, R. M., & Alexander, G. C. (2009). U.S. physician knowledge of the FDA-approved indications and evidence base for commonly prescribed drugs: Results of a national survey. *Pharmacoepidem. Drug Safe, 18,* 1094–1100.

Chow, S. C., & Chang, M. (2008). Adaptive design methods in clinical trials—A review. *Orphanet Journal of Rare Diseases, 3,* 11.

Deveaugh-Geiss, J., March, J., Shapiro, M., Andreason, P. J., Emslie, G., Ford, L. M., et al. (2006). Child and adolescent psychopharmacology in the new millennium: A workshop for academia, industry, and government. *Journal of the American Academy of Child & Adolescent Psychiatry, 45*(3), 261–270.

Fugh-Berman, A., & Ahari, S. (2007). Following the script: How drug reps make friends and influence doctors. *PLoS Medicine, 4*(4), e150.

Gibson, S. (2014). Regulating direct-to-consumer advertising of prescription drugs in the digital age. *Laws*, *3*, 410–438.

Government of Canada (R.S.C., 1985, c. F-27). Food and drugs act. Retrieved from http://laws-lois.justice.gc.ca/eng/acts/F-27/index.html.

Haw, C., & Stubbs, J. (2005). A survey of the off-label use of mood stabilizers in a large psychiatric hospital. *Journal of Psychopharmacology*, *19*(4), 402–407.

Howard, L., & Thornicroft, G. (2006). Patient preference randomised controlled trials in mental health research. *British Journal of Psychiatry*, *188*, 303–304.

Industry Canada. (2012). *Pharmaceutical industry profile*. Retrieved from http://www.ic.gc.ca/eic/site/lsg-pdsv.nsf/eng/h_hn01703.html.

Jepsen, P., Johnsen, S. P., Gillman, M. W., & Sørensen, H. T. (2004). Interpretation of observational studies. *Heart*, *90*(8), 956–960.

Krener, P., & Mancina, R. (1994). Informed consent or informed coercion? Decision-making in pediatric psychopharmacology. *Journal of Child and Adolescent Psychopharmacology*, *4*(3), 183–200.

Kuehn, B. M. (2010). Questionable antipsychotic prescribing remains common, despite serious risks. *JAMA*, *303*(16), 1582–1584. http://dx.doi.org/10.1001/jama.2010.453.

Larkin, I., Ang, D., Avorn, J., & Kesselheim, A. S. (2014). Restrictions on pharmaceutical detailing reduced off-label prescribing of antidepressants and antipsychotics in children. *Health Affairs*, *33*(6), 1014–1023.

Lavori, P. W., Rush, A. J., Wisniewski, S. R., Alpert, J., Fava, M., Kupfer, D. J., et al. (2001). Strengthening clinical effectiveness trials: Equipoise-stratified randomization. *Biological Psychiatry*, *50*(10), 792–801.

Leclerc, J. M., Laberge, N., & Marion, J. (2012). Metrics survey of industry-sponsored clinical trials in Canada and comparator jurisdictions between 2005 and 2010. *Health Care Policy*, *8*(2), 88–106.

Lenk, C., Koch, P., Zappel, H., & Wiesemann, C. (2009). Off-label, off-limits? Parental awareness and attitudes towards off-label use in pediatrics. *European Journal of Pediatrics*, *168*(12), 1473–1478.

March, J. S., Silva, S. G., Compton, S., Shapiro, M., Califf, R., & Krishnan, R. (2005). The case for practical clinical trials in psychiatry. *American Journal of Psychiatry*, *162*, 836–846.

Marks, D. M., Thanaseelan, J., & Pae, C. U. (2009). Innovations in clinical research design and conduct in psychiatry: Shifting to pragmatic approaches. *Psychiatry Investigation*, *6*(1), 1–6. http://dx.doi.org/10.4306/pi.2009.6.1.1.

McAllister, J. (2012). Trials and tribulations: Clinical trials: The national effort to attract more investments to Canada. *Health Research & Innovation Magazine*, (Winter), 14–18. Retrieved from http://www.healthcarecan.ca/st-in-service-of-health/special-initiatives/clinical-trials-summit-portal/.

Mintzes, B. (2005). *Educational initiatives for medical and pharmacy students about drug promotion: An international cross-sectional survey*. Geneva: World Health Organization/Health Action International. [WHO/PSM/PAR/2005.2]. Retrieved from http://www.haiweb.org.

Mintzes, B., Lexchin, J., Sutherland, J. M., Beaulieu, M. D., Wilkes, M. S., Durrieu, G., et al. (2013). Pharmaceutical sales representatives and patient safety: A comparative prospective study of information quality in Canada, France and the United States. *Journal of General Internal Medicine*, *28*(10), 1368–1375.

Morgan, S. G., Smolina, K., Mooney, D., Raymond, C., Bowen, M., Gorczynski, C., et al. (2013). *Canadian Rx Atlas: (The Canadian Prescription Drug Atlas)* (3rd ed.). Retrieved from the Centre for Health Services and Policy Research Website, http://www.chspr.ubc.ca.

Murphy, A. L., Gardner, D. M., Kisely, S., Cooke, C., Kutcher, S. P., & Hughes, J. (2013). Youth, caregiver, and prescriber experiences of antipsychotic-related weight gain. *ISRN Obesity, 2013*, Article ID 390130, 9 pages, http://dx.doi.org/10.1155/2013/390130.

Pharmaceutical Advertising Advisory Board. (2013). *Code of advertising acceptance*. Retrieved from http://www.paab.ca/paab-code.htm.

Pocock, S. J. (2003). The pros and cons of noninferiority trials. *Fundamental & Clinical Pharmacology, 17*(4), 483–490.

Rhee, J. (2009). The influence of the pharmaceutical industry on healthcare practitioners' prescribing habits. *The Internet Journal of Academic Physician Assistants, 7*(1), 1–7.

Rosoff, P. M., & Coleman, D. L. (2011). Case for legal regulation of physicians' off-label prescribing. *Notre Dame Law Review, 86*, 649.

Royal College of Psychiatrists. (2007). Use of licensed medicines for unlicensed applications in psychiatric practice (College report CR142). Retrieved from the Royal College of Psychiatrists Website http://www.rcpsych.ac.uk/files/pdfversion/cr142.pdf.

Salbu, S. R. (1999). Off-label use, prescription, and marketing of FDA-approved drugs: An assessment of legislative and regulatory policy. *The Journal of Law, Medicine & Ethics, 51*, 181.

Schachter, D. C., & Kleinman, I. (2004). Psychiatrists' attitudes about and informed consent practices for antipsychotics and tardive dyskinesia. *Psychiatric Services, 55*(6), 714–717.

Schachter, D., & Kleinman, I. (2006). Psychiatrists' documentation of informed consent: A representative survey. *Canadian Journal of Psychiatry, 51*(7), 438.

Senate's Standing Committee on Social Affairs, Science and Technology. (2012). *Canada's clinical trial infrastructure: A prescription for improved access to new medicines*. Retrieved from http://www.parl.gc.ca/Content/SEN/Committee/411/soci/dpk/01nov12/reports-e.htm.

Senate's Standing Committee on Social Affairs, Science and Technology. (2014). *Prescription pharmaceuticals in Canada: Off-label use*. Retrieved from http://senate-senat.ca/soci-e.asp.

Sibbald, B., & Roland, M. (1998). Understanding controlled trials. Why are randomised controlled trials important? *British Medical Journal, 316*(7126), 201.

Stallard, N. (2011). Group-sequential methods for adaptive seamless phase II/III clinical trials. *Journal of Biopharmaceutical Statistics, 21*(4), 787–801.

Sugarman, P., Mitchell, A., Frogley, C., Dickens, G. L., & Picchioni, M. (2013). Off-licence prescribing and regulation in psychiatry: Current challenges require a new model of governance. *Therapeutic Advances in Psychopharmacology, 3*(4), 233–243.

US Department of Justice. (2009). *Justice department announces largest health care fraud settlement in its history*. Retrieved from Office of Public Affairs Website http://www.justice.gov/opa/pr/justice-department-announces-largest-health-care-fraud-settlement-its-history.

US Department of Justice. (2010). *Pharmaceutical giant AstraZeneca to pay $520 million for off-label drug marketing*. Retrieved from Office of Public Affairs Website http://www.justice.gov/opa/pr/pharmaceutical-giant-astrazeneca-pay-520-million-label-drug-marketing.

US Department of Justice. (2013). *Johnson & Johnson to pay more than $2.2 billion to resolve criminal and civil investigations*. Retrieved from Office of Public Affairs Website http://www.justice.gov/opa/pr/johnson-johnson-pay-more-22-billion-resolve-criminal-and-civil-investigations.

Victora, C. G., Habicht, J. P., & Bryce, J. (2004). Evidence-based public health: Moving beyond randomized trials. *American Journal of Public Health, 94*(3), 400–405.

Virani, A. S., Bezchlibnyk-Butler, K., & Jeffries, J. J. (2011). *Clinical handbook of psychotropic drugs* (19th ed.). Cambridge, MA: Hogrefe & Huber Publishers.

Vogel, L. (2011). Boilerplate being tested for clinical trials. *Canadian Medical Association Journal, 183*(16), E1179.

Wazana, A. (2000). Physicians and the pharmaceutical industry: Is a gift ever just a gift? *JAMA*, *283*, 373–380.

West, S. G., Duan, N., Pequegnat, W., Gaist, P., Des Jarlais, D. C., Holtgrave, D., et al. (2008). Alternatives to the randomized controlled trial. *American Journal of Public Health*, *98*(8), 1359–1366.

Wilson, D. (2010). Side effects may include lawsuits. *The New York Times* (October 2), 3.

Appendix A

List of Online Resources

Availability of Online resources are subject to change. All web addresses listed here were available as of February 2015.

CHAPTER 1: INTRODUCTION

Peter Wall Institute for Advanced Studies, Canadian Working Group on Antipsychotic Use in Children report: http://www.childmeds.pwias.ubc.ca/sites/childmeds.pwias.ubc.ca/files/uploads_20

NeuroDevNet Inc.: http://www.neurodevnet.ca/

Canadian Paediatric Society: http://www.cps.ca/

University of British Columbia Therapeutics Initiative: http://www.ti.ubc.ca/

CHAPTER 2: PHARMACOEPIDEMIOLOGY OF ANTIPSYCHOTIC USE IN CANADIAN CHILDREN AND ADOLESCENTS

Center for Disease Control and Prevention: http://www.cdc.gov

CHAPTER 3: DO WE KNOW IF THEY WORK AND IF THEY ARE SAFE: SECOND-GENERATION ANTIPSYCHOTICS FOR TREATMENT OF AUTISM SPECTRUM DISORDERS AND DISRUPTIVE BEHAVIOR DISORDERS IN CHILDREN AND ADOLESCENTS

Facts for youth about mixing medicine, alcohol, and street drugs: http://drugcocktails.ca/

CHAPTER 4: ENSURING THE SAFETY OF CHILDREN TREATED WITH SECOND-GENERATION ANTIPSYCHOTICS

Diagnostic Screening Tools

General Practice Services Committee clinical and diagnostic screening tools and resources: www.gpscbc.ca/psp-learning/child-and-youth-mental-health/tools-resources

The Science and Ethics of Antipsychotic Use in Children. http://dx.doi.org/10.1016/B978-0-12-800016-8.09996-7

Height Measurements Resources

Guide to standard measurements for endocrine patients: http://www.bcchildrens.ca/NR/rdonlyres/8B924057-C0B5-4E07-8B35-7323BAA3F379/48840/endomeasure.pdf

Body Mass Index (BMI) Measurement Resources

Centers for Disease Control and Prevention, clinical growth charts: http://www.cdc.gov/growthcharts/clinical_charts.htm

World Health Organization, growth reference for children aged 5–19 years: http://www.who.int/growthref/who2007_bmi_for_age/en/

Physical Activity Resources

Canadian Society for Exercise Physiology guidelines: http://www.csep.ca/english/View.asp?x=587

Centers for Disease Control and Prevention, Adolescent and School Health resources: www.cdc.gov/healthyyouth

Healthy Diet Resources

Canada Food Guide Health Canada: http://www.hc-sc.gc.ca/fn-an/food-guide-aliment/index-eng.php

Canadian Diabetes Association: http://www.diabetes.ca/diabetes-and-you/healthy-living-resources/diet-nutrition/portion-guide

Public Health Agency of Canada healthy living: www.phac-aspc.gc.ca/hp-ps/hl-mvs/index-eng.php

Metabolic Monitoring Resources

CAMESA guidelines: http://camesaguideline.org

A Physician Handbook for Metabolic Monitoring for Youth with Mental Illness Treated with Second-Generation Antipsychotics: http://www.bcchildrens.ca/NR/rdonlyres/45697169-42E2-45E6-B870-0C1A8EC3C164/46605/metmonhb.pdf

Kelty Mental Health Resource Centre in British Columbia: http://keltymentalhealth.ca/toolkits, http://keltymentalhealth.ca/metabolic

BC Mental Health and Substance Use, metabolic monitoring program resources: http://www.bcmhsus.ca/resources/metabolic-program

CHAPTER 5: PEDIATRIC CLINICAL TRIAL ACTIVITY FOR ANTIPSYCHOTICS AND THE SHARING OF RESULTS: A COMPLEX ETHICAL LANDSCAPE

Health Canada's Clinical Trials Database: http://www.hc-sc.gc.ca/dhp-mps/prodpharma/databasdonclin/index-eng.php

International Clinical Trials Registry Platform, World Health Organization: http://www.who.int/ictrp/en/

StaR Child Health (International Forum of Standards for Research in Children): http://ifsrc.org/

Tri-Counsel Policy Statement, 2nd edition, for the ethical conduct of research involving humans: http://www.pre.ethics.gc.ca/eng/policy-politique/initiatives/tcps2-eptc2/Default/

Canadian Clinical Trials Coordinating Centre: http://www.cctcc.ca/

Drug Products Database: http://webprod5.hc-sc.gc.ca/dpd-bdpp/

CHAPTER 6: PATHWAYS TO OVERMEDICATION AND POLYPHARMACY: CASE EXAMPLES FROM ADOLESCENTS WITH FETAL ALCOHOL SPECTRUM DISORDERS

Children's Sleep Network: http://www.childrenssleepnetwork.org/WP/

Canadian Pharmacogenomics Network for Drug Safety (CPNDS): http://www.cpnds.ubc.ca/

CHAPTER 7: IMPLEMENTING CHANGE IN PRESCRIBING PRACTICES

School curriculum resources: http://teenmentalhealth.org/curriculum/

Canadian Agency for Drugs and Technologies in Health Rx for Change database: http://www.cadth.ca/en/resources/rx-for-change/database

CHAPTER 8: CANADIAN INITIATIVES AND RECOMMENDATIONS: SAFEGUARDING THE HEALTH OF CHILDREN AND YOUTH RECEIVING OFF-LABEL TREATMENT WITH ANTIPSYCHOTICS

Canadian Adverse Reaction Newsletter: http://www.hc-sc.gc.ca/dhp-mps/medeff/bulletin/index-eng.php

Canadian Paediatric Surveillance Program (CPSP), ADR Tips of the Month: http://www.cpsp.cps.ca/publications/adr-tips-of-the-month

Protecting Canadians from Unsafe Drugs Act (Vanessa's Law), Amendments to the Food and Drugs Act (Bill C-17), Health Canada: http://www.hc-sc.gc.ca/dhp-mps/legislation/unsafedrugs-droguesdangereuses-eng.php

Canada Health Infoway: https://www.infoway-inforoute.ca/

Maternal Infant Child, Youth Research Network (MICYRN): http://www.micyrn.ca/

Canadian Institutes of Health Research, Drug Safety and Effectiveness Network: http://www.cihr-irsc.gc.ca/e/40269.html

Index

Note: Page numbers followed by *f* indicate figures and *t* indicate tables.

A

Aberrant Behavior Checklist (ABC), 49
Aberrant Behavior Checklist-Irritability
    subscale (ABC-I), 51
Abnormal involuntary movement scale (AIMS)
    scale, 50
Accreditation Canada, 176–177
ADHD. *See* Attention-deficit/hyperactivity
    disorder (ADHD)
Adverse drug reactions (ADRs), 176
  case study, 134–137
  informed consent, for patients and
    caregivers, 178
  prevalence, 127–128
  reporting process, 177–178
American Psychiatric Association Choosing
    Wisely campaign, 164–165
Antipsychotics, 149
  academic clinical trials, 96, 101*t*
  active clinical trials, 96, 97*t*
  American Psychiatric Association Choosing
    Wisely campaign, 164–165
  aripiprazole, 5
  behavior change techniques, 165–170, 167*t*
  collaborative clinical trials, 96, 101*t*
  COM-B assessment and intervention
    functions, 163, 163*t*
  completed clinical trials, 96, 97*t*
  decision making, 152–153
  discontinued clinical trials, 96, 97*t*
  expansion, 4–6
  factors influencing prescribing decisions,
    152–153, 153*f*
  patient-physician relationships, 170
  pharmaceutical clinical trials, 96, 101*t*
  pragmatic approach, 149–150
  prescribers, 150–151
  school environment, 155
Applied behavioral analysis (ABA) therapy, 51
Aripiprazole, 5, 14–15, 28, 57, 117–118
Artificial hibernation, 1–2
ASDs. *See* Autism spectrum disorders (ASDs)
Attention-deficit/hyperactivity disorder (ADHD)
  disruptive behavior disorders, 29
  drug prescriptions, guidelines for, 140–141
  medications, 140–141

  second-generation antipsychotic
    recommendations, 16–17, 17*f*
Autism spectrum disorders (ASDs). *See also*
    Second-generation antipsychotics (SGAs)
  ABC-I subscale, 51
  adverse effects and safety data, 54–56
  applied behavioral analysis, 51
  aripiprazole, 31
  efficacy, trials, 57–58
  flexible-dose design, 50–51
  Gilliam Autism Rating Scale, 52
  intellectual disability, 31–50
  olanzapine, 31
  RCTs, 31, 32*t*

B

Barnes Akathisia rating scale (BARS), 50
BCTs. *See* Behavior change techniques (BCTs)
BCW. *See* Behavior change wheel (BCW)
Behavioral adverse drug reactions (ADRs),
    127–128, 142–143
Behavior change techniques (BCTs), 167*t*
  Dynamic Sustainability Framework,
    169–170, 169*f*
  guideline-concordant monitoring,
    166–169
  illness-and medication-related
    objectives, 166
  and intervention functions, 165–166
  program drift and voltage drop, 166–169, 168*f*
  selection of, 165
Behavior change wheel (BCW), 162–163, 162*f*
Best Pharmaceuticals for Children Act
    (BPCA), 28, 93
Blood pressure, 76
Body mass index (BMI), 55, 76
British Columbia Ministry of Health
    PharmaNet database, 21–22

C

Canada Health Infoway, 177–178
Canada's Compendium of Pharmaceuticals and
    Specialties (CPS), 190
Canada's Drug Safety and Effectiveness
    Network (DSEN), 182, 183

Canadian Adverse Reaction Newsletter (CARN), 176–177
Canadian Alliance for Monitoring Effectiveness and Safety of Antipsychotics in Children (CAMESA), 69–73
Canadian clinical trials
  action plan recommendations, 182
  design strategies, 183, 184*t*
  randomized control trials, 183
  research and development, 181
  sales revenue loss, 181, 182
Canadian Clinical Trials Coordinating Centre (CCTCC), 93–94
Canadian health care system, mechanisms in, 150
Canadian Paediatric Surveillance Program (CPSP), 176
Canadian pharmaceutical marketing regulatory policies, 183–187
  educating about marketing strategies, 189–191
  industry regulation, 187–189
  PAAB guidelines, 189
Canadian SGA prescription trends, 15
Capability, opportunity, motivation–behavior (COM-B)
  assessment, 161–162
  description, 160–161
  schematic illustration, 161*f*
CFIR. *See* Consolidated Framework for Implementation Research (CFIR)
Childhood Autism Rating Scale (CARS), 49, 52
Child Mania Rating Scale (CMRS) tool, 49, 53–54
Children's Global Assessment Scale (CGAS), 52
Children's Yale-Brown Obsessive-Compulsive Scale (cY-BOCS) tool, 49
Chlorpromazine, 1–2, 3
Citalopram, 16
Clinical Global Impressions (CGI) scale, 49, 109
The Clinical Handbook of Psychotropic Drugs, 190
Clozapine, 4, 56
The Cochrane Database of Systematic Reviews, 190
COM-B. *See* Capability, opportunity, motivation–behavior (COM-B)
The Compendium of Therapeutic Choices, 190
Consolidated Framework for Implementation Research (CFIR)

guidelines, 159–160
implementation factors, 158
prescribing behavior change, 160, 161*t*
schematic illustration, 159*f*
cY-BOCS tool. *See* Children's Yale-Brown Obsessive-Compulsive Scale (cY-BOCS) tool

D

Daytime-focused medication cascades, 138
Disruptive behavior disorders (DBDs). *See also* Second-generation antipsychotics (SGAs)
  ABC-social withdrawal/lethargy subscale, 54
  adverse effects and safety data, 54–56
  aripiprazole, 53–54
  efficacy, trials, 58
  flexible-dose design, 53
  intelligence quotient, 53
  methylphenidate, 53
  quetiapine, 53–54
  RCTs, 39*t*, 52
  visual analog scale, 54
Disruptive mood dysregulation disorder (DMDD), 28
Drug discontinuation design, 30
Dynamic Sustainability Framework, 169*f*

E

Electronic medical record (EMR), 177–178

F

FASDs. *See* Fetal alcohol spectrum disorders (FASDs)
FDA Cosmetic Act of 1938, 92–93
Fetal alcohol spectrum disorders (FASDs)
  description, 125–126
  overmedication and polypharmacy, 127–128
  patient demographics, 129, 130*t*
  in pediatric patients, 128–134
  prescription and medication practices, 129, 131*t*, 134
  prevalence rates, 125–126
  sleep problems, 127
Fluoxetine, 16

G

Gilliam Autism Rating Scale (GARS), 52, 57

H

Harris-Kefauver Amendment, 92–93
Health Canada, 4–5
  adverse drug reaction, 176, 177
  aripiprazole, 28
  drug safety, 176–177
  Pediatric Expert Advisory Committee, 182
Health monitoring, SGAs, 68–69
Hyperkinetic syndrome, 22
Hypnagogic hallucinations, 141–142

I

Industry Practices Review Committee, 187–188
Informed consent process
  barriers, 179–180
  in minor patients, 179–180
  patient autonomy, 178
  standardized patient consent form, 179

K

Kelty Mental Health Resource Centre, 84–85

L

Lifesaving anticancer drugs, 6
Life Trajectory Chart, 135, 136f

M

Manitoba Health Drug Program Information Network database, 18
Maternal Infant Child, Youth Research Network (MICYRN), 182
Melatonin, 139–140
Metabolic complications management
  diet modification, 79–80
  lower-risk agent, 78
  lowest effective dose, 78
  polypharmacy reduction, 80
  regular physical activity, 79
Metabolic monitoring tool (MMT), 69–73, 70f
Methylphenidate, 16

N

Neurodevelopmental conditions, pediatric sleep problems, 126–127
Nisonger Child Behavior Rating Form (N-CBRF), 49
Non-pharmacological interventions, 121

O

Off-label antipsychotic prescriptions, 121, 175
  artificial hibernation, 1–2
  benefits, 6–8
  Canadian pharmaceutical marketing regulatory policies, 183–191
  children, 4–6
  clinical trials, 180–183
  guidelines for, 191–192
  informed consent
    barriers, 179–180
    in minor patients, 179–180
    patient autonomy, 178
    standardized patient consent form, 179
  partnership, 8–9
  post-approval monitoring of, 176–178
  psychopharmacology research, 2–3
  quinine, 1
  reporting adverse events, 176–177
  second-generation antipsychotics, 3–4
Olanzapine, 15

P

Parasomnias, 135
Parent/caretaker influence, in decision-making process, 154
Patient care, 81–82
Patient safety, 92–93
Pediatric clinical trial activity, antipsychotics
  Canadian Clinical Trials Coordinating Centre, 93–94
  clinical trial registration, 94
  clinical trial regulation, 92–93
  developmental gaps, 113–114
  ethics, 92–93
  FDA-approved drugs, 116–117
  informed consent, 119
  landscape, 112–113
  limitations, 120
  methods, 95–96
  outcome measures, 116
  patient safety, 92–93
  peer-review process, 117
  pharmaceutical industry trials, 117
  psychiatric conditions, 91–92
  recommendations, 120–121
  recruitment and willingness, research, 118–119
  registry databases, 92
  results, 96–112
  strength of evidence, 114–116
  Tri-Council Policy Statement, 94–95
  U.S. FDA Modernization Act, 93
  World Health Assembly, 93–94
  World Medical Association, 94–95

Pediatric Research Equity Act (PREA), 93
Pharmaceutical Advertising Advisory Board
  (PAAB), 189
Pharmacoepidemiology
  British Columbia, 21–22
  Manitoba, 18–19
  medication use assessment, 13
  national prescribing trends, 15–18
  Nova Scotia, 19–20
  SGAs (*see* Second-generation antipsychotics
    (SGAs))
Pharmacotherapeutic decision making,
  150–153
PharmaNet, 177–178
Polypharmacy, 126
Prenatal substance exposure (PSE)
  medication history in pediatric patients,
    128–134
  patient demographics, 129, 130*t*
  prescription and medication practices, 129,
    131*t*, 134
Prescribing behavior change frameworks
  behavior change wheel, 162–163, 162*f*
  CFIR, 158, 159–160, 159*f*
  COM-B, 160–162, 161*f*, 161*t*
  schematic illustration, 157, 158*f*
Prescription drugs, 125–126
PRISMA diagram, 30, 30*f*, 31*f*
PSE. *See* Prenatal substance exposure (PSE)
Psychiatric care, decision-making approach
  in, 152
Psychopharmacology research, 2–3
Psychostimulants, 140–141
Psychotropic decision making
  prescriber experience of, 155–157
  youth and family experience of, 153–155

Q
Quality of Life Enjoyment & Satisfaction
  Questionnaire (Q-LES-Q), 53–54
Quetiapine, 16
Quinine, 1

R
Randomized controlled trials (RCTs)
  ASDs, 31, 32*t*
  Canadian clinical trials, 183
  critique and ethical considerations, 59–60
  DBDs, 39*t*, 52
  second-generation antipsychotics, 56
Relatively informed decision-making model, 152

Restless legs syndrome. *See* Willis Ekbom
  disease (WED)
Risperidone, 15, 16, 19

S
Schizophrenia, decision-making approach in,
  152
Second-generation antipsychotics (SGAs),
  138, 141–142
  active family engagement, 82
  aripiprazole, 28, 65–66
  ASDs (*see* Autism spectrum disorders
    (ASDs))
  atypical/dopamine-serotonin
    antagonists, 13
  barriers, metabolic monitoring, 82–85
  Best Pharmaceuticals for Children Act, 28
  blood pressure, 76
  body mass index, 76
  Canada *vs.* other countries, 14–15, 22–23
  Canadian prescription trends, 15
  disruptive mood dysregulation disorder, 28
  FDA-approved indications, 65–66, 66*t*
  fever of child psychiatry, 29
  guidelines, metabolic monitoring, 69–73
  health monitoring, 68–69
  height, 73
  long-term effects, 66–67
  mental health disorders, 67
  metabolic complications management,
    76–81
  metabolic monitoring protocol, 65–66, 74*t*
  metabolic side effects, 13–14
  methods, 29–56
  patient care, 81–82
  RCTs, 56
  side effects, 67–68
  waist circumference, 76
  weight, 76
Self-awareness, 153–154
Sensory processing abnormalities, 138–139
SGAs. *See* Second-generation antipsychotics
  (SGAs)
Shared decision-making model, 152
Simpson Angus Scale (SAS), 50
Sleep problems
  day/nighttime presentations, 141, 141*f*
  fetal alcohol spectrum disorders, 127
  in pediatric patients, 128–134
  therapeutic emplotment, 143
  videosomnography, 143
Standardized patient consent form, 179

T

Therapeutics Initiative (TI), 7, 190–191
Traditional decision-making medical model,
    152

U

U.S. FDA Modernization Act, 93

V

Vanessa's Law, 176–177

W

WED. *See* Willis Ekbom disease (WED)
WHO International Clinical Trials Registry
    Platform policy, 94

Willis Ekbom disease (WED)
    case study, 134–137
    diagnosis, 138–139
    gabapentin treatment, 139
    prevalence, 127

Y

Young Mania Rating Scale (YMRS), 53–54,
    109